T0137431

Studies in Systems, Decision and Control

Volume 123

Series editor

Janusz Kacprzyk, Polish Academy of Sciences, Warsaw, Poland
e-mail: kacprzyk@ibspan.waw.pl

About this Series

The series "Studies in Systems, Decision and Control" (SSDC) covers both new developments and advances, as well as the state of the art, in the various areas of broadly perceived systems, decision making and control- quickly, up to date and with a high quality. The intent is to cover the theory, applications, and perspectives on the state of the art and future developments relevant to systems, decision making, control, complex processes and related areas, as embedded in the fields of engineering, computer science, physics, economics, social and life sciences, as well as the paradigms and methodologies behind them. The series contains monographs, textbooks, lecture notes and edited volumes in systems, decision making and control spanning the areas of Cyber-Physical Systems, Autonomous Systems, Sensor Networks, Control Systems, Energy Systems, Automotive Systems, Biological Systems, Vehicular Networking and Connected Vehicles, Aerospace Systems, Automation, Manufacturing, Smart Grids, Nonlinear Systems, Power Systems, Robotics, Social Systems, Economic Systems and other. Of particular value to both the contributors and the readership are the short publication timeframe and the world-wide distribution and exposure which enable both a wide and rapid dissemination of research output.

More information about this series at http://www.springer.com/series/13304

David E. Forbes · Pornpit Wongthongtham
Chamonix Terblanche · Udsanee Pakdeetrakulwong

Ontology Engineering Applications in Healthcare and Workforce Management Systems

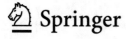
Springer

David E. Forbes
Independent Researcher
Perth, WA
Australia

Chamonix Terblanche
City of Cockburn
Perth, WA
Australia

Pornpit Wongthongtham
Curtin University
Perth, WA
Australia

Udsanee Pakdeetrakulwong
Nakhon Pathom Rajabhat University
Nakhon Pathom
Thailand

ISSN 2198-4182   ISSN 2198-4190   (electronic)
Studies in Systems, Decision and Control
ISBN 978-3-319-87925-3   ISBN 978-3-319-65012-8   (eBook)
DOI 10.1007/978-3-319-65012-8

Printed on acid-free paper

This Springer imprint is published by Springer Nature
The registered company is Springer International Publishing AG
The registered company address is: Gewerbestrasse 11, 6330 Cham, Switzerland

Preface

The exponential growth of demand for sharing of knowledge beyond the normative mental capacity of human beings is accelerating construction of and contributions to the Semantic Web. Development and integration of computer ontologies, with multi-agent knowledge access systems serving both related and disparate domains of value to society, have become vital imperatives in the opening decades of the twenty-first century. This book builds upon separate research activities simultaneously conducted between 2009 and 2013. It examines and promotes the merging for purpose, of two ontology concepts while including an update review of both domains. Employer Demand Intelligence (EDI) signifies articulation of methods for projecting worker needs, while Patient Practitioner Assistive Communication (PPAC) offers a pathway to a more productive engagement between patients and healthcare practitioners, notably involving culturally and linguistically disadvantaged patient communities. In concert and with philosophical justification, these two ontology concepts are presented as formulaic ontology propositions for the introduction of efficiencies in the critical supply chain for evolving and future healthcare delivery.

Chapter 1 **Current Issues**
The first chapter introduces the conceptual ecosystem for knowledge management modelling. Three key questions about discovery, data and change parameters are posed and discussed. Current issues are supported with a general overview of trends emerging over the last few years with emphasis on change affecting the two domains; most significantly affecting Employer Demand Intelligence as illustrated by contemporary and emerging disruptive influences in recruitment processes.

Chapter 2 **Information Technology Challenges and Opportunities**
Expansion of the world of data and accompanying digital enterprise complexity as research and development activity brings new opportunities and challenges. Big Data, Data Analytics, Data Science and Disruptive Technology are covered in context. Emphasis is placed on greater awareness of advances in artificial intelligence and machine learning, and importance of interdisciplinary research.

Multi-agent system (MAS) advantages are explored with explanation of Agent Communication Language (ACL) message exchange.

Chapter 3 Ontology Engineering

This chapter presents domain knowledge representation and organisation via specific structure(s). It focuses on ontology engineering methodologies, ontology design, ontology editor tool and reuse of existing ontologies. There is no single consensual ontology engineering methodology. Examination of some is given to illustrate the differences. Six different ontology engineering methodologies are covered and compared. Protégé editor tool and logical consistency verification are explained.

Chapter 4 Patient Practitioner Assistive Communication Ontology

This chapter specifies development of the Patient Practitioner Assistive Communication (PPAC) ontology. It briefly covers all PPAC ontology classes and subclasses, properties and constraints, with future access to fine detailed development. Graphics include Type 2 Diabetes Ontology Concepts; Aboriginal English Home Talk Ontology Concepts; Object and Data Properties; ontology instance populations. Text contains a case study in which distinctive cultural attributes are then accommodated in the ontology structure.

Chapter 5 Cross-Cultural Healthcare Communication System

This chapter follows on from the previous chapter presenting healthcare communication systems in which the PPAC ontology and knowledge base are placed as main components. It presents data and knowledge assimilation in and dissimilation from the PPAC ontology. It illustrates the system architecture and considers components, knowledge capture, knowledge linking and integration, and anticipation of continued growth with expansion of knowledge. A practical use case scenario is offered.

Chapter 6 Employer Demand Ontology

This chapter is to crossover to the workforce management topic. It presents development of Employer Demand Ontology (EDO)-based Application for employer demand identification with EDO. Concepts are divided into two parts, i.e. non-specific job advertisements and detailed occupation-specific. Overview of EDO as developed in Web Ontology Language (OWL), EDO classes and Object and Data Properties is presented. Case scenario relating to Government Official Developing Policy and Funding Protocols is covered. It shows querying and its result illustrated from Protégé system. Vacancy advertisements, Human Resources management and tertiary training make up three case scenarios.

Chapter 7 Employer Demand Intelligence

This chapter emphasises the importance of job market status clarity. It introduces Employer Demand Intelligence Tool (EDIT), with system architecture, unstructured and structured data collection description and case scenario. It specifically focuses on occupations under the Registered Nurse and Midwifery classification. Seven-step process in EDIT Pipeline is presented.

Chapter 8 **Intelligent System**

This chapter correlates domains including software engineering, health, education, e-commerce, finance, etc. and provides a summary of existing ontology-based multi-agent systems. Literature review of MAS is presented. It covers integration of Ontologies and Software Agents, ontology for knowledge representation, knowledge integration, knowledge sharing and reuse. Software agent and multi-agent system are for benefits of autonomy, reactivity, pro-activeness, social ability, adaptability and dynamism. Employment Demands and Healthcare Service Delivery Management Systems are discussed in combination with questions still to consider: factoring in uncertainty affecting physicians' perspectives and confidence; study of implications for culturally competent critical healthcare staffing; and cognitive computing. It also includes a vector-borne infectious disease epidemic case study.

Chapter 9 **Open Issue and Concluding Remarks**

This chapter merges issues and relationships embracing Employment and Service Communications; shared knowledge weaknesses; western medical culture power distance; unsatisfactory healthcare worker communications; patients disadvantaged due to lack of cultural competence; and disease symptom diagnosis and treatment controversies that also influence communications. It also includes Multicultural Mental Health Australia (MHiMA) project data illustrating cultural and linguistic diversity in Australia. It offers advocacy concept for blending of EDI and Culturally Competent Health Care (CCHC) domain ontologies.

Perth, Australia   David E. Forbes
Perth, Australia   Pornpit Wongthongtham
Perth, Australia   Chamonix Terblanche
Nakhon Pathom, Thailand   Udsanee Pakdeetrakulwong

Contents

Acronyms

ACL	Agent Communication Language
ACT	Assistive Communications Technology
AE	Aboriginal English
BDA	Big Data Analytics
CALD	Culturally and Linguistically Diverse
CFS	Chronic Fatigue Syndrome
DL	Description Logic
EDI	Employer Demand Intelligence
EDO	Employer Demand Ontology
GPs	General Practitioners
HR	Human Resources
ICT	Information, Communications and Technology
KS	Knowledge Sharing
KT	Knowledge Transfer
MAS	Multi-Agent System
ME	Myalgic Encephalomyelitis
MUS	Medically Unexplained Symptoms
PPAC	Patient Practitioner Assistive Communication
PPIEs	Patient Practitioner Interview Encounters
RDF	Resource Description Framework
SM	Social Media
SPARQL	SPARQL Protocol and RDF Query Language
T2DM	Type 2 Diabetes Mellitus
URIs	Uniform Resource Identifiers

Chapter 1
Current Issues

1.1 Introduction

This book is designed to provide a philosophical perspective brief on what may be regarded as a conceptual ecosystem as an example of information systems and knowledge management modelling. We aim to cover employer demand intelligence (EDI) and patient practitioner assistive communication (PPAC) concepts and the cross-over factors among them. This is not an exhaustive process. It retains the researcher spirit for the works to embrace and to accommodate thoughts about future prospects. Contemplating the future is to think about change. Discovery, data and change go hand in hand. Questions to take are as follows:

- What has changed in the (Australian) world of employee recruitment manifested in EDI methods and systems?
- What changes have occurred in cross-cultural healthcare communications, most specifically relating to patient practitioner interview encounters with Australia's Aboriginal community Type 2 diabetes patients?
- What appears to be the activity driven by system developments affecting either or both of the research domains?

In this chapter, current issues and a general overview of the related and published trends emerging over the last few years in the two domains are provided.

1.2 Recruitment Practices Changing

The dynamics of changing recruitment practices; from advertising, interviewing and selection to the time of employment of candidates, have become distinct by the speed and versatility of web based options. The Australian Government Job Search

© Springer International Publishing AG 2018
D.E. Forbes et al., *Ontology Engineering Applications in Healthcare and Workforce Management Systems*, Studies in Systems, Decision and Control 123, DOI 10.1007/978-3-319-65012-8_1

website posting of December 2015 invited visitors to contemplate how their business strategy compares with the most popular recruitment methods in Australia. The survey data drawn from 10,000 employers showed that 48% of all vacancies that are advertised are placed on the internet, with 18% representing the declining trend, placed in newspapers. Around half of the latter are also advertised on the internet. The report also advised that one third of jobs are not formally advertised (Meet the Most Popular Recruitment Methods in Australia 2015).

Molly Green (2015) offered advice on getting jobs that are never advertised. From considerable talent acquisition and Human Resources (HR) experience, (Molly Green 2015) asserted that the landscape has changed dramatically over the past 3–5 years but without firm validation, it is estimated that 80% of jobs filled come from the hidden jobs market, that is, those that are not advertised.

We have witnessed an increase in the mining of employer demand intelligence related data, as stated by McLean et al. (2016). Data protection/privacy laws in Asia, Europe and North America present potential legal liabilities. When identifying keywords and concepts for a data collection exercise, organizations need to apply the same rigor that they would use when creating job advertisements. This is particularly pertinent for the use of automated data collection and decision making systems.

The term employer branding, although not enjoying a common definition, is widely viewed as the creation of organizational attractiveness, and is a marketing concept designed as much as for any other business purpose to optimize appeal and serious interest on the part of potential and talented employees whom the organization wishes to target. Several authors have explored the development and popularity of this pre-recruitment strategy (Lean et al. 2015; Alnıaçık et al. 2014; Hinojosa et al. 2015). To some extent, accepting the constant technology driven shifting of practices among and between employer and potential employee sectors, we may justifiably perceive this as a form of reverse engineering. Using another analogy there are signs that there is increased fishing and filtering being conducted by job-seekers as opposed to search and selection domination by employing organizations.

For its part HR at the professional level is indirectly as well as directly influential in the recruitment process. Almost as an extension or appendage to the employer branding strategy, promoting sustainability within an organisation is gradually being recognised as beneficial to recruitment. Jepsen and Grob (2015) offered a framework of sustainability practices. From a listing of ten recommendations we include here three practices which we judge represent interactive potential for enhanced demand intelligence (Jepsen and Grob 2015):

- Paperless processes. Using technology to reduce paperwork is perhaps the most environmentally preferable practice.
- Recruitment from within.
- Flexibility to encourage applicant diversity.

The first of these points includes reference to now frequent electronically-conducted recruitment multi-faceted communications processes. The second qualifies the point by stating that a reputation for developing personal growth opportunities for its own employees is more likely to make it an employer of choice. Lastly, applying variable hours and being more amenable to accommodate dissimilar applicant group types such as older, disabled, physically distant and other minority workers should improve the scoping value of job advertisements.

These three dimensions can be embodied in practical applications by first identifying conversationally engaging terminology in the contemporary candidate market context. Social media (SM) platforms such as Facebook, LinkedIn, Twitter etc. are sources of emerging words, phrases and the communications style preferences of SM visitors, subscribers and article bloggers. Within specific workgroup cultures, sector-unique terminologies and acronyms can become obstacles to a flexible and successful talent search. Recruitment from within is one source for rectifying this weakness, by helping to build the electronic linguistics and context bridge to elevate demand intelligence value.

In a discussion about future recruitment processes, and specifically organizational culture as key elements of the hiring process, (Ghinea 2015) pointed out the weaknesses within work cultures that sometimes results in the hiring of an under-qualified or over-qualified person. Whereas recruitment is commonly a positive exercise, in contrast the subsequent selection process is a negative one (Ghinea 2015). This then hints at the absence of good 'employer branding' of the organization. Moreover, and as a reminder of trends in employee loyalty and independence, no company buys the applicant; it just rents their abilities and knowledge. This has the subtle effect of indicating where power shifts occur in employment and in recruitment processes; and by inference, how recruiter perceptions, aided by employee retention trend data, can identify qualitative gaps in demand intelligence. 'Demand intelligence' in this sense refers not to an exclusive employer controlled domain of influence but to a broader meaning, effectively the sharing of 'demand' between job vacancy owner and the candidate pool 'marketplace'.

Based upon employment research in Cyprus, the use of social network sites as an e-recruitment tool is reported (Melanthiou et al. 2015). From Facebook Key Facts (2013), United States Census Bureau (2014), today about one in every six individuals maintain a social network profile on Facebook, while one in every 28 own LinkedIn accounts. Melanthiou et al. (2015) Illustrated the push and pull power shift; we are told that 'e-recruitment is a fast-growing method of employees as more and more individuals post their résumés online in search for a better future'. Although there appears to be an as yet unquantifiable mix and fluctuation between employer-candidate demand initiative sources, there is concern about legal liability and data trustworthiness in the SM ecosystem. The authors remind us that published e-recruitment related research articles date back no more than a decade; and that most emanate from American and European studies involving large organisations. They propose further investigation to explore the e-recruitment process through the eyes of the applicant adding that Information is scarce regarding applicant expectations and reception, especially during a newly created strategy such as e-recruitment.

Uma and Praveen (2015) promote the use of multi agents as having significant value for elaborating the job description, getting applicants to submit competencies relevant to the job advertised, shortlisting of candidates and ultimately identifying 'the right hire'. We note in particular the reference to 'competencies', reinforcing the qualitative measure implicit within a merged ontology serving the recruitment skill, experience and qualification needs in cross-cultural healthcare delivery. Educational institutions need to take greater note of and adjust to contemporary measures; responding to the impact of lag time between what researchers are able to report through drawn out publications processes, and the topicality of other web generated sources of demand intelligence factors. Our literature review has tended to show that the 'blogger sphere' and higher end social media platforms are dictating the pace of change, leading the way for higher education to follow, to tap into through the use of Big Data Analytics (BDA) software tools, and thereby build more knowledge sharing information systems and social communications immediacy into business school curricula.

There are no agreed standards for knowledge sharing in existence today; and the private entity platforms appear to be exploiting this with their 'disruptive', competitive, entrepreneurial incursions.

These authors characterised a virtual intelligent agent as an autonomous entity that can make intelligent conversations and negotiation with one or more virtual human agents in a specific domain. They also make some salient points about the 21st Century employee candidate search process. The technological changes make it hard to ensure that HR personnel are current and capable in the context of knowledge of and in both technical and non-technical sectors. Training, retention and growth of employees, again reflecting an employer's historical workforce management reputation, are seen as contributing to the volatility of the contemporary recruitment scene. The authors then resort to a proposal for the development of an intelligent agent system to accommodate customization of a résumé for a specific job application. A consequential benefit from this system is the facilitation of priority ranking on the part of the employer in the interview scheduling phase. It is suggested in this paper that this will prove to be most effective within a professional online network such as LinkedIn.

Talent Board is an American based non-profit organisation promoting and data-benchmarking qualitative research into the experience of engagement from the candidate population perspective. Published survey results are produced annually. The key findings are summarised as follows (Talent Board Reveals 2015 North American Candidate Experience Research 2016).

- More sophisticated candidates: Candidates continue to take more control of their own journey; 76% conduct their own job search research across multiple channels prior to applying.
- Onboarding becomes automated: More employers are leveraging onboarding solutions, with more than 60% using technology to automate forms management.

- Interviews become more efficient: Employers are conducting fewer interviews per candidate, with 79% of companies now having one or two interviews related to a position, compared to 63% in 2014.
- Mobile apply is still lagging: Although many technology providers have improved or enhanced their mobile capabilities, companies that offer mobile apply only see 8–10% of their candidates applying through a mobile device.
- Candidate communication can be improved: Although most companies send an immediate automated "thank you," nearly half of all candidates never receive an indication of the status of the application, and overall candidate communication has decreased from the application process to screening and dispositioning when compared to the 2014 CandE Research.

A 2015 United Kingdom study into the Candidate Experience of 2013 in that country states three pillars of candidate attraction and an employer's ability to convert employment prospects into candidates are: (1) Online channels, (2) Content and (3) Transparency (The Candidate Experience Report 2015).

Posing a question about effectiveness of employers' online strategies, this report reveals that candidates were queried on the ways they accessed information about the potential 'target' employer. The response indicated that online tool investment by employing organisations is justified by the evidence that when such channels are available they are accessed regularly. Specifically, the common online channels are: the Company's Career Site, Career Site Agents, LinkedIn Company Pages and Facebook Career Pages.

Among the bloggers and debaters about present and future employment prospects, there are sceptics who point to unsatisfactory or unreliable job statistics (O'Brien 2014). Employment Outlook reports emphasize lagging skills transition, stronger job-search obligations and serious concerns about vulnerable youth impacted by poor employment prospects (OECD 2016). Routine media reports about job advertisements are also indicators of demand (Workplace Info 2016). The unpredictable nature, the employer and worker impact of uncertainty in this immense social transition has commonly invoked and provoked serious intellectual thought about change. This quite commonly surfaces as phenomena described variously as industry disruption, or technological disruption, suggesting a strong reliance on innovative entrepreneurial and initial adoption of uncomfortable non-traditional ways of doing things.

One potentially disruptive innovative for-profit talent scoping and management software organisation trading as PageUp, in its commercial offerings addresses the need for improved understanding by employing organisations of 'the lag between job seeker demand and the execution of employer mobile strategies'. In a study of Australia's one hundred largest companies the PageUp research report shows six key findings (New Study from PageUp Finds Australia's Top Employers Too Slow to Embrace Mobile Technology in Recruitment 2015):

- Overall, nearly 40% of career sites studies provided a poor search experience and more than one-quarter had no online application process. These companies have effectively taken themselves out of the race to secure talent.
- Nearly three-quarters of Australia's largest companies lack mobile-optimised career sites and approximately two-thirds of career sites only have basic functionality.
- Only half of the top 100 companies use social referrals to reach untapped talent, and only 40% enable job seekers to receive job alerts. This represents a missed opportunity to engage candidates and maximise their talent pipelines.
- Less than half of the career sites (45%) allow candidates to pre-populate their application form from social media profiles and resumes, which can significantly speed up the process.
- More than a quarter of companies (29%) inadvertently reduce their candidate pool by half because their career site is not compatible with iOS devices, such as iPads and iPhones.
- Only one-third of career sites can tap the entire talent pool by allowing candidates to attach resumes from cloud storage—a unique vendor-specific functionality offered by PageUp ensuring candidates can apply regardless of which device they use.

It is arguable, and we conditionally support this point, that the activities of bloggers and social media subscribers provide a more contemporary picture of trends in multiple knowledge streams, when compared with the protracted process in which peer-reviewed research publications eventually reach interested reviewers. Moreover, academic research output is not commonly read, digested and directly acted upon by the general public. The primary audience is made up from the primary peer group specialist interests. Notwithstanding the absence of consistent peer-review and accompanying quality assurance disciplines, worthy and frequently creative, imaginative material is found on the Web and originates from entities and individuals with a genuine ethical intent in sharing data and interpretation, albeit frequently with commercial objectives. Given the apparent suddenness of technologically innovative product and service disruption impacts, it appears wise to respect the potential value of web-based data sources outside of the academic research realm. The import of accepting this approach to decision-making is at times a partial shift from a majority reliance on peer-review research publication; imposing the quality assurance due-diligence evaluation trust-quotient activity and ultimate judgement on the end-user cohort.

In a commercial opinion, (Lucas 2016) asked the question "Is the recruitment industry about to be disrupted?". The author claims that over the last fifteen years the recruitment industry has effectively 'played' with new business models that promised disruption, without sustained success. Describing the industry pressures, Google has been called 'the great disruptor', largely based upon rumours about its intention to relaunch the recruitment platform known as 'Google Base'. After excluding indifferent performance by specialised industry job boards as low-value economy he points to one successful exception, i.e. LinkedIn. In the new players' entry discussion, the blog article goes into the disruptive incursion by non-traditional recruiting sources, i.e. technology companies that are not intrinsically HR specialists or recruitment agency businesses. Challenges are coming from well-funded successful start-ups that have the skill, resources and money.

In similar vein, (Marcum 2016) observed the diminishing value of older algorithms in recruitment systems that operate on single platforms and the overwhelming HR weight of searching through a high volume of candidate profiles, while wading through many that are outdated and describe people no longer seeking work. Filter techniques such as keyword criteria devised to optimise candidate application and inquiry complexities appear to present efficiency gains. But discussing the promise of Artificial Intelligence in employer demand intelligence, Marcum opens up the 'flip-side' with cautionary advice about reducing and thereby risking the harm of losing the personable aspect of candidate engagement (Marcum 2016).

LinkedIn is an omnipresent social media career professionals-oriented networking platform with global reach. (Abbot et al. 2016) developed its fifth of a series of annual reports with the data content and analysis derived from a survey of 3894 'talent acquisition decision makers'. Relevant key findings from the perspective of detecting influencers and trends in employer demand intelligence are extracted and listed here (Abbot et al. 2016):

Most important trends

- 26% consider employee referral programs to be a long-lasting trend
- 59% are investing more in their employer brand compared to last year

Obstacles to attracting top talent:

- 46% Finding candidates in high demand talent pools
- 43% Compensation
- 39% Competition

Referrals grow as a key source of quality hires—sources compared

- 43% Social professional networks
- 42% Internet job boards
- 32% Employee referral programs (up from 26% in 2015)

Recruiting trends to keep in mind (Organisational intent—Looking ahead)

- 39% Utilizing social and professional networks
- 38% Employer branding
- 28% Finding better ways to source passive candidates
- 26% Employee referral programs.

1.3   Patient-Centred Communications

For the last few years, there has been a lack of focused capability, political will and consequential patient-centred communications in the Australian healthcare environment and other developed countries. There are few models which help to remedy cross-cultural communications barriers using the advantages of assistive communications technology (ACT). The ACT potential after all is a derivative of successful established and increasingly popular mass market applications available on a variety of mobile devices. It is somewhat ironic that we are able to develop prioritize and sell communications systems for routine remote conversation, texting and audio-visual content sharing, meeting the high demand for entertainment; yet using the same technology in a patient-centred consultation context to support physical and mental wellbeing and to sustain our quality of life and enjoyment of these benefits, falls far short as a comparative investment.

The worrying epidemiological picture of the Type 2 Diabetes Mellitus (T2DM) chronic illness is persisting across the world. Obesity in developed countries and the high related risk of developing T2DM is cause for alarm when we consider the educated and relatively sophisticated healthcare knowledge sharing opportunities present in 21st Century Australasia, Europe and North America.

It is noted that communications weaknesses, mostly at the cost of patient understanding, cooperation and wellbeing, are often present in Patient-Practitioner Interview Encounters (PPIEs) regardless of the cultural origin of the patient. The research acknowledges the decision making cognitive engagement barrier of an authoritative power-based medical culture; and the relative educational distance between patient and practitioner, in particular adversely affecting people from disadvantaged backgrounds and/or communities. This is far reaching and of considerable consequence to healthcare services in countries trying to cope with immigrant communities from very different cultures than that of the host state.

Forbes (2013) was focused on the extraordinary incidence and prevalence of Type 2 Diabetes (T2DM) chronic disease affecting Australia's Aboriginal and Torres Strait Island (ATSI) population. Intercultural communications barriers impose adverse impacts on a much broader population. A country with large numbers of migrants from non-English speaking nations, and an unknown portion of the Australian born descendants from similar cultures, stands to gain much in the world of healthcare and medical research. Cultural competence is essential for successful engagement with culturally and linguistically disadvantaged groups, who regardless of ethnicity may also include Australians suffering from disabilities or from educational disadvantage. With this desirable inclusivity factor in mind, we contend that the ontology based technological developments which we advocate are of considerable social value, within and beyond Australia's shores. Moreover by implication, investment in or neglect of, improved healthcare communications will find their respective worth in epidemiological outcomes, including the cost of healthcare service delivery. Among the ultimate benefits from provision of machine supported intelligent culturally-competent communications systems is reduction of hospitalizations and consequential costs of same arising from failed understanding in the primary care setting.

NA (2015) summarized dissatisfaction with the disappointing outcomes of a program initiated in 2008. The article briefly refers to the withdrawal of essential services in Western Australia and the significant impact on health and wellbeing of remote living Aboriginal people effectively forced to move from their traditional land in order to receive health care services.

Reilly (2015) reported on the findings of the fourth annual 'Broadband for the Bush Forum' held in Darwin. Much focus was given to the call for "alternative last-mile delivery options" for communities, taking account of Wi-Fi access, and emphasizing support for essential services including healthcare; and specifically overcoming remote telecommunications, data caps and internet connection black-spots. Recognizing Australia's increasing reliance on online services support, the forum warned that absence of flexibility will lead to a failure in closing the digital divide between urban and remote Australia.

Wang et al. (2016) were addressing the increasing complexity of large scale interdisciplinary research projects commonly established to foster cross-disciplinary cooperation and to utilize potential synergies. The Collaborative Research Center (CRC) project examined 19 individual projects from different disciplines to evaluate perspectives and solutions for sustainable manufacturing. The authors observe that research activities require the creation of a shared understanding for which task a common CRC ontology should be developed. They explain simply that an ontology can serve as a unifying framework to solve problems regarding communication between persons and/or organizations (e.g. by providing a normative model), interoperability (e.g. by enabling re-use and sharing of data/information/models between IT-systems), and systems engineering (Wang et al. 2016).

Working toward information infrastructure (INF) the findings from this project disclosed many challenges for integrating data management across disciplines, ranging from copyright obstacles, the generation and inclusion of raw data, confidentiality concerns, among a large list of issues to overcome. This article elaborates more fully on the R&D essentials to be confronted i.e. to ensure long-term preservation and availability of research data and that more persistent infrastructures such as institutional repository services from university libraries should be utilized.

1.4   Assistive Communications Technology

Assistive communications technology (ACT) has been introduced, used, and is being developed as a healthcare support tool. In context, it is not too great an expectation that in a time that has seen tremendous efficiency advances in such systems as cell-phone products and services, and in social media knowledge sharing, chronic disease patients should see simultaneous gains in the quality and effectiveness of portable healthcare communications software and devices.

A demonstrable paucity of discussion about ACT has been identified within the published research articles, implicitly suggesting that the 'digital divide' is more than a remote and disadvantaged community communications progress barrier. It illustrates the contemporary weakness of healthcare practitioners and researchers to purposefully embrace inter-disciplinary research into and thereby keep pace with the broader societal communications momenta. Titles examined which within their claimed research discourse are intended to improve primary care patient support have been disappointingly lacking in even the basics of technological insight.

Works that are devoid of the role of ACTs include as follows. Towards better preparation and support for health and social care practitioners (Lindeman et al. 2014), the role of primary health care services better meet the needs of Aboriginal Australian transitioning from prison to the community (Lloyd et al. 2015). Health literacy especially in the oral exchange is an important element of patient-provider communication (Nouri and Rudd 2014). Exploring the relationships between participatory decision-making, visit duration, and general practitioners provisions argumentation to support their medical advice (Labrie and Schulz 2015). Baba et al. (2014) studied into how Indigenous services address health impacts of discrimination. Mohammad et al. (2015) investigated exploration of culturally diverse consumer needs for medicine use and health within pharmacy settings.

The foregoing contrasts with the impressive investment in Australia's medical technology as discussed and featured in Medical Technology in Australia: Key Facts and Figures (2014). The word 'paucity' so often used by researchers when explaining gaps in research output and knowledge can however be explained by many dimensions that are in play outside of academic research. These include willingness of technology companies to support new concepts; the existence at any time of commercially sensitive products and services in the modelling phase necessitating secrecy for intellectual property protection. Most demanding of the challenge is complexity arising from the exponential algorithmic need to merge and match ontologies; and intelligent agent integration so that the communications regimen is accurate, robust and perpetually capable of growing in step with sustainable, reliable, culturally competent patient-centred healthcare conversation lexicology. Mobile applications related to healthcare do exist but not in the context of PPIE ACTs designed to overcome intercultural or other forms of patient disadvantage disparities in primary care communications.

This gap in ACT implementation and the barriers or delay mechanism just described is further exacerbated by weakness in the appreciation by medical service providers of the patient-centred priority for much better understanding from the knowledge sharing exercise that is inherent but too often lost within PPIEs. Simplistically we refer to this as the cultural communications bridge or lingua franca. The cost of a lack of understanding translates among other things, to excessive but not necessarily successful consumption of time, instead of time-saving, which is one of the key attractions for ACT. Brandes et al. (2014) studied the barriers to expressing concerns during cancer consultations. Succinctly the authors point to the temporal dimension, i.e. time. Results showed that the most influential barriers were related to providers' behaviour (e.g. providers do not explicitly invite patients to express concerns) and the environment where the consultation takes place (e.g. perceived lack of time) Brandes et al. (2014).The authors however did not explore ACT supportive options.

Asan et al. (2014) used video recordings to assess how physicians' electronic health record screen sharing affects communication in PPIEs. The conclusion of this paper is motivating. The healthcare system in the US is moving from a paternalistic model to a more egalitarian approach that focuses on patients' preferences, needs, and values (i.e. patient-centered care) to optimize outcomes (Asan et al. 2014). The authors point out that research is underway to show how the presence of computers in the consultation room affects patients. A similar paper, again more focused on physician computer usage and knowledge, is offered by Sobral et al. (2015). Our perspective from these articles is that this may be a small step in moving toward wider use of ACTs, in which the patient data will have a life outside of the consulting room; and also managed by the patient or representative groups outside of government.

Lloyd (2014) posed the question: How do Resettling Refugees Connect with Health Information in Regional Landscapes? Lloyd (2014) addressed implications for health literacy in the Australian context as follows:

- Barriers: Cognitive, social and structural barriers
- Cultural beliefs and Information
- Adapting to a different health culture
- Information overload
- Conceptions of health literacy.

These aptly describe the data and interpretative capture domains for ACTs but the author's remit rests with health literacy barriers and does not move toward the social media or technology role in helping refugees connect with health information.

Some hope of higher value in the ACT adoption context comes from O'Mara (2014). The paper took qualitative research project findings involving communities from Vietnamese, Sudanese and Samoan backgrounds all living in the west part of Melbourne. Without actually presenting a proposed course of development, (O'Mara 2014) hypothesized that a major issue is generic and top-down health communication which does not engage effectively with culturally and linguistically diverse populations. New and emerging forms of information technology (IT) can help address this problem and disparities in aged care through more inclusive forms of communication. Smartphones, web sites, social media, video conferencing and other IT are being used to create tailored and user friendly health content, as well as interactive, participatory and community-driven online environments for supporting access to health services, including with aged community members (O'Mara 2014).

Further papers/publications reviewed extend the discussion but these have tended to be written in the tone of 'what must be done' versus 'what we are doing about it'. There are dozens of sources falling under that descriptive category. Alexander et al. (2015) looked at prejudices and perceptions of patient acceptance of mobile technology use in health care. The authors acknowledge the rapidly transforming health care setting in the image sense and evidence of health professionals multitasking and interacting with smartphones. Although the technology revolution is well advanced, apart from research into use of personal digital assistants, few studies have evaluated patient and family perceptions of the use of mobile devices (smartphones and tablets) by qualified or student health professionals at the patient bedside in hospital settings (Alexander et al. 2015). The paper reported on a 2013 evaluation study in an adult and paediatric teaching hospital in Sydney; with seventy patients and their carers participating. Whereas the main topic was the use of devices by medical staff, and familiarity with mobile communications devices provides understanding of the benefits and some tolerance of professionals using them in the consultation setting, one third of those surveyed expressed a dislike for the practice by doctors of using mobile devices at the bedside. In the closing remarks, this paper also effectively reinforces the importance of integrity within the communications domain. Bringing together the comment about limited evaluations of the patient community viewpoint; acknowledging the inference that having rapidly adopted mobile phone use without seeking the patient community opinion, that healthcare providers are not even entertaining the equitable possibilities of patient empowered use of mobile devices, the authors draw attention to a call for codes of conduct. Potential distraction, lack of etiquette and risk of security and privacy breaches are important issues that need to be addressed if those working in the healthcare environment are to embrace fully mobile technology as we progress further into the 21st century. Changes in practice stemming from the increasing ease of access to knowledge and practitioners bring with it calls for new codes of conduct, which need to be respected by all. Patient education may also be needed to ensure qualified and student health professionals of all disciplines are able to use mobile devices to improve the effectiveness of their work.

1.5   Conclusion

This book describes cross-cultural healthcare concepts and employer demand intelligent concepts. We aim to transcend two hitherto unconnected and dissimilar domains by investigating the cross-over factors. In this first chapter, we presented issues around recruitment practices changing, patient centric communications, and assistive communication technology. Literature in the areas have been specified covering related and published emerging trends. In the next chapter, challenges and opportunities in information technology will be presented.

References

Abbot, L., Batty, R., Bevegn, S.: Global Recruiting Trends 2016 - Relationships at the Core. (2016)

Alexander, S.M., Nerminathan, A., Harrison, A., Phelps, M., Scott, K.M.: Prejudices and perceptions: patient acceptance of mobile technology use in health care. Intern. Med. J. **45**, 1179–1181 (2015). doi:10.1111/imj.12899

Alnıaçık, E., Alnıaçık, Ü., Erat, S., Akçin, K.:. attracting talented employees to the company: do we need different employer branding strategies in different cultures? 10th International Strategic Management Conference 2014. In: Proceedings Social and Behavioral Sciences: 10th International Strategic Management Conference 2014 **150**, 336–44. doi:http://dx.doi.org/10.1016/j.sbspro.2014.09.074 (2014)

Asan, O., Young, H.N., Chewning, B., Montague E.: How physician electronic health record screen sharing affects patient and doctor non-verbal communication in primary care. Patient Educ. Couns. **98**, 310–16 (2014). doi:http://dx.doi.org/10.1016/j.pec.2014.11.024

Baba, J.T., Brolan, C.E., Hill, P.S.: Aboriginal medical services cure more than illness: a qualitative study of how indigenous services address the health impacts of discrimination in brisbane communities. Int. J. Equity Health **13**, 1–10 (2014). doi:10.1186/1475-9276-13-56

Brandes, K., Linn, A.J., Smit, E.G., van Weert., J.C.M.: Patients' reports of barriers to expressing concerns during cancer consultations. Patient Educ. Couns. **98**, 317–22 (2014). doi:http://dx.doi.org/10.1016/j.pec.2014.11.021

Facebook Key Facts. Statistics. Available at http://newsroom.fb.com/Key-Facts (2013). Accessed 11 May 2016

Forbes, D.E.: A Framework for Assistive Communications Technology in Cross-Cultural Healthcare. Curtin University (2013)

Ghinea, V.M.: Filling present vacancies by means of future oriented recruitment processes. Proceedings in Manufacturing Systems **10**(1), 29–38 (2015)

Hinojosa, A.S., Walker, H.J., Payne, G.T.: Prerecruitment organizational perceptions and recruitment website information processing. Int. J. Hum. Resour. Manag. **26**, 2617–2631 (2015). doi:10.1080/09585192.2014.1003081

Jepsen, D.M., Grob, S.: Sustainability in recruitment and selection: building a framework of practices. J. Educ. Sustain. Dev. **9**(September), 160–178 (2015). doi:10.1177/0973408215588250

Labrie, N.H.M., Schulz, P.J.: Exploring the relationships between participatory decision-making, visit duration, and general practitioners provision of argumentation to support their medical advice: results from a content analysis. Patient Educ. Couns. **98**, 572–77 (2015). doi:http://dx.doi.org/10.1016/j.pec.2015.01.017

Lean, H.H., Saleh, N.M., Sohail, M.S., Ahmad, N.A., Daud, S.: Engaging People with Employer Branding. In: Proceedings Economics and Finance: 7th International Economics & Business Management Conference (IEBMC 2015) **35**, 690–98 (2015). doi:http://dx.doi.org/10.1016/S2212-5671(16)00086-1

Lindeman, M., Dingwall, K., Bell, D.: Towards better preparation and support for health and social care practitioners conducting specialised assessments in remote indigenous contexts. Aust. J. Soc. Issues **49**, 445–465 (2014)

Lloyd, A.: Building information resilience: how do resettling refugees connect with health information in regional landscapes—Implications for health literacy. Aust. Acad. Res. Libr. **45**, 48–66 (2014). doi:10.1080/00048623.2014.884916

Lloyd, J.E., Delaney-Thiele, D., Abbott, P., Baldry, E., McEntyre, E., Reath, J., Indig, D., Sherwood, J., Harris, M.F.: The role of primary health care services to better meet the needs of aboriginal Australians transitioning from prison to the community. BMC Fam. Pract. **16**, 1–10 (2015). doi:10.1186/s12875-015-0303-0

Lucas, P.: Is the recruitment industry about to be disrupted? Blog. Available at http://www.akqire.
    com.au/Perspectives/2016/07/19/Is-the-Recruitment-Industry-about-to-Be-Disrupted/   (2016).
    Accessed 11 Dec 2016

Marcum, B.: Why Artificial Intelligence Will Disrupt the Recruiting Industry. Available at https://
    kandktechnical.com/artificial-intelligence-will-disrupt-recruiting-industry/ (2016). Accessed 6
    Oct 2016

McLean, S., Stakim, C., Timner, H., Lyon, C.: BIG data and human resources: letting the
    computer decide? Scitech Lawyer **12**, 20–23 (2016)

Medical Technology in Australia: Key Facts and Figures 2014. Available at http://www.mtaa.org.
    au/Docs/Key-Documents/Facts-Figures_final-Website-Version.pdf (2014). Occasional Paper
    Series. Medical Technology Association of Australia, Sydney. Accessed 5 Jun 2016

Meet the Most Popular Recruitment Methods in Australia: How Does Your Strategy Compare?
    Australian Government JobSearch Website Posted 10/12/2015 https://Jobsearch.gov.au/Most-
    Popular-Recruitment-Australia/Default.aspx (2015). Accessed 31 Aug 2016

Melanthiou, Y., Pavlou, F., Constantinou, E.: The use of social network sites as an e-recruitment
    tool. J. Trans. Manag. **20**, 31–49 (2015). doi:10.1080/15475778.2015.998141

Mohammad, A., Saini, B., Chaar, B.B.: Exploring culturally and linguistically diverse consumer
    needs in relation to medicines use and health information within the pharmacy setting. Res.
    Soc. Adm. Pharm. **11**, 545–59. (2015) doi:http://dx.doi.org/10.1016/j.sapharm.2014.11.002

Molly Green.: How to get the jobs that are never advertised. Available at http://www.lifehacker.
    com.au/2015/11/How-to-Get-the-Jobs-That-Are-Never-Advertised/ (2015) Accessed 5 May
    2016. *Lifehacker*

NA.: Aboriginal Healthcare: Closing the Gap—Another Year of Failure. Available athttp://search.
    informit.com.au/documentSummary;dn=101237063261532;res=IELHEAMedicus **55** (2015).
    Accessed 6 Jun 2016

New Study from PageUp Finds Australia's Top Employers Too Slow to Embrace Mobile
    Technology in Recruitment. Available athttps://www.pageuppeople.com/en-sg/news_item/
    australias-top-employers-too-slow-to-embrace-mobile-technology-in-recruitment-rec001/ (2015).
    Accessed 15 Feb 2016

Nouri, S.S., Rudd, R.E.: Health literacy in the oral exchange: an important element of patient
    provider communication. Patient Educ. Couns. **98**, 565–71 (2014). doi:http://dx.doi.org/10.
    1016/j.pec.2014.12.002

O'Brien.: Why Job Figures Are Failing Us. Available at http://www.charteredaccountants.com.au/
    News-Media/Charter/Charter-Articles/Economy/2014-05-Why-Job-Figures-Are-Failing-Us.aspx
    (2014). Accessed Aug 2016

OECD.: OECD Employment Outlook 2016. OECD Publishing (2016)

O'Mara, B.: Aged care, cultural and linguistic diversity and it in Australia: a critical perspective.
    Int. J. Migr. Health Soc. Care **10**, 73–87 (2014)

Reilly, C.: Remote Communities Call for Digital Inclusion in Outback Australia. Available at
    https://www.cnet.com/Au/News/Remote-Communities-Call-for-Digital-Inclusion-at-Broadband-
    for-the-Bush-Forum/ (2015). Accessed 7 May 2016

Sobral, D., Rosenbaum, M., Figueiredo-Braga, M.: Computer use in primary care and
    patient-physician communication. Patient Educ. Couns. **98**, 1568–76 (2015). doi:http://dx.
    doi.org/10.1016/j.pec.2015.07.002

Talent Board Reveals 2015 North American Candidate Experience Research: New Report
    Highlights the Latest Trends and Proven Strategies to Deliver an Exceptional Candidate
    Experience Press Release. Available at http://www.thetalentboard.org/Press-Releases/Talent-
    Board-Reveals-2015-North-American-Candidate-Experience-Research/ (2016). Accessed 12
    Dec 2016

The Candidate Experience Report 2014. Available at http://www.kellyservices.co.uk/
    uploadedFiles/United_Kingdom_-_Kelly_Services/New_Smart_Content/Business_Resource_
    Center/Talent_Acquisition/CandE_Research_Paper_2014_FINAL.pdf (2015). Kelly Services
    UK. London Accessed 12 Mar 2016

Uma, G., Praveen, P.: (HR)^2: An agent for helping hr with recruitment. Int. J. Agent Technol. Sys. (IJATS) **7**, 67–85 (2015). doi:10.4018/ijats.2015070104

United States Census Bureau.: U.S. and World Population Clock. https://www.census.gov/popclock (2017). Accessed 5 Jan 2017

Wang, W.M., Göpfert, T., Stark, R.: Data management in collaborative interdisciplinary research projects—Conclusions from the digitalization of research in sustainable manufacturing. ISPRS Int. J. Geo-Inf. **5** (2016) doi:10.3390/ijgi5040041

Workplace Info: Job Ads Fell in September. Available at https://workplaceinfo.com.au/recruitment/news/job-ads-fell-in-september (2016). Accessed 5 Dec 2016

Chapter 2
Information Technology Challenges and Opportunities

2.1 Introduction

In the last decade, the world of data and digital enterprise has expanded, becoming greatly enriched but also more complex as research and development activity continues to introduce new opportunities and challenges across the spectrum of human educational endeavour. Usage of descriptive words and phrases including titles such as Big Data, Data Analytics, Data Science and Disruptive Technology are commonplace within the information, communications and technology (ICT) field. Some of these terms have existed for decades; the frequency of their appearance however, notably in online publications and social media content, denotes the catalytic coincidence of greater awareness of the potency of exponential strides in the advancement toward artificial intelligence and machine learning. Collectively the label Big Data or BDA is capturing attention in the commercial sphere, particularly in the context of companies that use technology and continuous machine-supported development to enhance efficiencies in financial services delivery. The term widely adopted in this process is 'FinTech' (Wikipedia 2016).

In the build-up to this point, knowledge transfer (KT) defined by King (2010) as 'any exchange of knowledge between or among individuals, teams, groups, or organizations, whether intended or unintended' emphasizes both the vital capacity of the human brain to exchange, digest and analyse information and the feeding or conversion of that information into knowledge. King and He, in a separate book chapter to that referenced earlier, write about Knowledge Sharing (KS) as distinct from Knowledge Transfer, describing KS in the context of organisational assets intended to achieve commercially competitive advantage (King and Jun He 2010). Avoiding the trap of entering into the distinctions and varied definitions offered about knowledge transfer and knowledge sharing we are concerned in this book to encourage collaboration across disciplines, supported through continuous development of machine-based data management and analytical capabilities. Pre-occupation with definitions can cause some distraction for research authors; and

© Springer International Publishing AG 2018
D.E. Forbes et al., *Ontology Engineering Applications in Healthcare and Workforce Management Systems*, Studies in Systems, Decision and Control 123, DOI 10.1007/978-3-319-65012-8_2

the KT/KS example is accompanied with various terms used to describe coopera-
tive activities across mixed research specialisms, i.e. Cross-disciplinary,
Interdisciplinary, Multidisciplinary and Transdisciplinary. A common characteristic
emerging from these similar terms is the intentional move away from the constraints
of an often attributed silo mentality in academic research institutions.

2.2   Interdisciplinary Research

Without playing a game of favourites and contributing to an unnecessary debate, we
choose to use the term 'Interdisciplinary research' (IR) which we deem for the
purposes of this book as the integration and value-output delivery processes
emerging from research into disparate domain concepts, the data and their relationships. There are innumerable permutations of such integrations. Pohl et al.
(2015) have explored the challenges of publishing IR, looking at hindrance and
support factors. Scholars finding it difficult to publish interdisciplinary research
complain of the lack of journal reviewers who place value on IR. In Pohl et al.
(2015), a sociologist who posed a question about how to collaborate with a biol-
ogist, stating "What should we write about? I don't know".

A specialist subject researcher such as in a healthcare-specific domain may need
to translate technical data relationships and properties into lay-consumer language
in order to support a mobile communications device application serving the particular patient community. Calling upon expert source material then amounts to
cross-disciplinary research activity. But it does not necessarily contribute to a
reciprocal exchange of information. It is KT and primarily a one-way process. Put
simply we need information to help build the knowledge base. In a mutually
symbiotic exchange, anticipating KS, interdisciplinary research represents a transition from the cross-disciplinary KT status, denoting joint enterprise and some
form of shared return from the research investment, financial or non-financial.
Again put simply, but in this new context, we need to share information to help
build and enrich the knowledge base in which we enjoy a mutual research interest.

2.3   Semantic Web and Linked Data

2.3.1   Semantic Web

The Semantic Web is an extension of the World Wide Web in which the meaning or
semantics of information and services is defined (Campbell and MacNeill 2010),
making it possible for people as well as machines to "understand" the web content.
In essence, it makes a shift for data modelling not only in human readable but also
machine readable format. This means that machines are capable of semantic

processing and reasoning. Since the Semantic Web term appeared in the early 2000s, a large amount of research has been done resulting in a number of publications in the area.

The fundamental building block playing a significant role in the semantic web is the Resource Description Framework (RDF). The meaning is expressed by RDF encoded in the form of subject—predicate—object expressions also known as triples.

2.3.2 Linked Data

Linked Data refers to a collection of interrelated data (Campbell and MacNeill 2010). It lies at the heart of the semantic web. This concept has gained traction after the publication of large Semantic Web resources such as DBPedia, Bio2RDF, etc., and by the announcement by some Governments of their decision to make public data public, in a set of Open Government initiatives e.g., data.gov, data.gov.uk (Heath and Bizer 2011). DBPedia makes the Wikipedia data and other datasets e.g. Geonames, available in RDF. By providing those links within and between the datasets, it allows applications to exploit knowledge from datasets (Campbell and MacNeill 2010).

Linked data provides a way to publish data on the semantic web that encourages reuse, reduced redundancy, maximises its interconnectedness, and enables network effects in order to add value to data (Heath and Bizer 2011). Berners-Lee (2009) states that in principle, linked data uses Uniform Resource Identifiers (URIs) as names for things and uses HTTP URIs so that people can look up those names. When a URI is found through SPARQL (a recursive acronym for SPARQL Protocol and RDF Query Language), it provides useful RDF information and includes RDF statements that link to other URIs so that they can discover more things.

2.3.3 Challenges and Opportunities

The semantic web makes search processes easier for finding, sharing, reusing and integrating information; effectively helping to interpret and convert information so that it takes on a knowledge status value. The quality of data found in the semantic web is not however self-evident when considered at the datum level, i.e. as a singular piece of information. Correlations of data drawing upon different semantic web search sources present the opportunity to move toward acceptance that data outputs are reliable; but for significantly sophisticated exercise, size and density limit the productivity of the collation process and its intended benefits.

The vast, inestimable volume of data and its constant rapid growth dominated through the worldwide web 'super-library', and by accessibility to extensive data base resources, defy any human solo or team opportunity to cognitively capture all of the pertinent datasets for acquiring sufficient knowledge to successfully address a specific-topic problem. The additional barrier to such knowledge acquisition or 'capture', is the complexity of the data and the relationships that exist or may potentially exist, in them. Identification of relationships within and developmentally possible for data therefore demands a cross-disciplinary exchange capability. Education in its fundamental form is a knowledge transfer activity. Purposeful interactions between individuals and entities increasingly demand the sharing of knowledge between two or more, and more frequently today, multiple, subject matter domains.

Taxonomies, nomenclature, and contextual interpretation for the most part unique to subject matter domain ecosystems, present educational obstacles and knowledge transfer opportunities. The processes for and productive outcomes from, cross-disciplinary research and collaboration are at the human cognition level burdened with labour intensive, time consuming and cultural compatibility challenges.

2.4   Ontologies as Building Blocks for the Semantic Web

The key foundations of the Semantic Web are ontologies. Ontologies, which are normally represented in the RDF Schema or Ontology Web Language (OWL), describe formally shared conceptualizations of a domain of interest (Gruber 1993).

Solodovnik (2010) described the concept of Ontology from its philosophical origins to its adoption within the ICT field as follow:

> Philosophically, Ontology is a systematic explanation of being that describes the features of Reality. Nowadays Ontology is proliferating in organizing Knowledge of different domains managed by advanced computer tools. Ontology qualifies and relates semantic categories, dragging, however, the idea of what, since the seventeenth century, was a way to organize and classify objects in the world. Ontology maximizes the reusability and interoperability of concepts, capturing new Knowledge within the most granular levels of information representation. Ontology is subjected to a continuous process of exploration, formation of hypothesis, testing and review. Ontological thesis proposed today as true, tomorrow may be rejected in light of further discoveries and new and better arguments.

The growth of ontologies has tended to be based upon specification of concepts with dedicated topics with limited work directed toward cross-pollination of knowledge and know-how. As this book brings together two seemingly discordant domains, we perceive this as an opportunity to prompt researchers and ontologists to seek new models for machine learning systems.

We consider how societal need-based probabilities will emerge from interactive domain data possibilities. While at first sight EDI and ACT in Cross-Cultural Healthcare Communications (CCHC) occupy distinctly different domains comprised of disparate data, ontology supported knowledge development and management for societal progress present considerable KS enrichment opportunities. In the interdisciplinary research mode and with good cause such as commercial market opportunities, the ontologies representing these two ostensibly unconnected domains represent potentially rewarding exploitation prospects. Bridging the functionality and resultant KS gap between these two ontologies (for example) offers enhancement of the intellectual capabilities in a third, combined, domain, i.e. cross-cultural recruitment communications processes for the healthcare sector. Australia depends on healthy net immigration flows to continue to build and sustain its intellectual and economic future.

The use of machine support systems increases the potential of the value factor through greater resource efficiencies. This is attractive to serious researchers for several reasons. Speed and accuracy for the collection and management of complex data will facilitate justifiable confidence to ameliorate the research delivery model. The research constraints touched upon in the previous section can be mitigated through task devolution techniques which employ ontology construct principles. Ontology development offers the benefit of emulation of human collaboration by capturing and employing interdisciplinary research precepts (Wang et al. 2016).

In a human conversation, the two domains in simpler terms (employer recruitment healthcare communication) can be easily assimilated. They are very common facets of contemporary life and social discourse in the developed world.

Why and how might we bring about the coalescence of diverse domain knowledge as a machine learning and intelligent machine reasoning capability? The term 'Artificial Intelligence' (AI) emerges from this thought process. AI however may not reliably convey the objectives or the 'ultimate goal' of advancing ontology constructs. A 2004 paper on computational ontologies and information systems lists 'artificial intelligence, knowledge representation, information science, library science, and database management' as matters 'of inquiry, development and application' (Kishore et al. 2004).

Indicative of the ontology and machine learning fields of research, we find reason these several years on, to refine our thinking and intentions about AI in particular. We nevertheless advocate for the continual evolution of intelligent machine systems for which ontologies will play a significant productive role as the building blocks for machine learning and for machine-independent simulation of human brain power and ensuing capabilities. In this closer examination of the goal of intelligent machines, we commonly find mischaracterizations, largely arising from fascination in the form of speculative media articles about robotics, threats to human labour from automation and science fiction entertainment depictions of AI. Kelly (2015) provided some informative relief from the 'AI fiction' obsession. Kelly (2015) asserts that the future of intelligent systems technology will be 'cognitive' as opposed to 'artificial'. They generate not only answers to numerical problems but also hypotheses, reasoned arguments and recommendations about more complex and meaningful bodies of data. Cognitive systems can make sense of the 80% of the world's unstructured data. This enables them to keep pace with the volume, complexity and unpredictability of information and systems in the modern world.

2.5   Agent-Based Technology

Agent-based technology has attracted substantial attention and has become an active research area in recent years. In addition, the advent of the Semantic Web technology has provided the underlying infrastructure that allows software agents to process data and perform sophisticated tasks on behalf of users. A definition of term 'agent' that has been widely accepted is given by Wooldridge (2009):

> An agent is a computer system that is situated in some environment and that is capable of autonomous action in this environment in order to meet its delegated objectives.

According to Wooldridge and Jennings (1995), Jennings (2000), the key properties of an agent are as follows.

- Autonomy: agents encapsulate some state and make decisions on what to do based on this state without the direct intervention of humans or others.
- Reactivity: agents are situated in an environment and are able to perceive this environment through their sensors. Then, through effectors, they respond in a timely fashion to changes that occur in their environment.
- Pro-activeness: agents do not simply act in response to their environment. They are able to exhibit goal-directed behaviour by taking the initiative.
- Social ability: agents are able to cooperate with humans and other agents in order to achieve their design objectives.

Software agents can be differentiated from traditional software applications in terms of certain characteristics. The differences between traditional software applications and software agents are presented in Table 2.1.

Table 2.1 Differences between traditional software applications and software agents, adapted from Turban et al. (2010)

Characteristics	Traditional software applications	Software agents
Nature	Static	Dynamic
Autonomy	Follow instructions	Be able to perform tasks without direct control, or at least with the minimum of human intervention
Manipulation	User initiates every action	Sense the environment and react autonomously
Interactivity	Non-interactivity	Can interact with other agents, humans, or software programs
Temporal continuity	Terminate when process is complete	Continue to run over time (persistent)
Concurrency	Generate process in one dedicated server with limited processing power	Dispatch simultaneously to accomplish several parts of a task in parallel
Mobility	Stay in one place	Be able to travel from one machine to another

From Table 2.1, it is clear that the software agents are different from traditional software applications. Moreover, compared with the object-oriented paradigm, the agent technology can be considered as a descendant that improves the nature of passive objects with the notion of autonomous actors (Braubach et al. 2005). In contrast to simple objects with methods that can be invoked by other objects, an agent communicates with other agents by means of message-passing. In addition, it can act proactively to accomplish its individual goal. Agents can work as stand-alone entities to perform particular tasks on behalf of a user. However, many agent applications are based on environments that contain multiple agents collaboratively working together as a group. This is also known as a multi-agent system.

Even though an individual agent can perform a task on behalf of a single user, its capacity is limited by its knowledge and resources. Thus, agents are usually implemented in a multi-agent context. A multi-agent system (MAS) consists of multiple agents acting in an environment to achieve a common goal or their individual goals (Ye et al. 2016). There is an increasing interest in MAS research because of its significant advantages including its ability to solve problems that may be too large for a single agent. MAS allows a complex task to be decomposed into subtasks, each of which is then assigned to an individual agent to undertake independently, but which can be supported by a knowledge base. They have distributed architectures which control distribution by utilising the mechanisms of cooperation and coordination.

MAS have various advantages over a single agent, such as reliability and robustness, modularity, scalability, adaptability, concurrency, parallelism, and dynamism (Elamy 2005). When a system is implemented based on MAS architecture, it is easy to add a new functionality or to modify an existing functionality. Within MAS, the functionality is created by calling the service that a particular agent offers. Therefore, in order to add a new functionality, a new agent responsible for a new service can be added into a system. In order to modify or improve the functionality of the system, the existing agent can be modified or substituted with a new one. In this case, a system is loosely coupled which means that it is easy to extend, remove, and modify without breaking down the system. In addition, MAS can make the system more fault-tolerant by replacing an agent that has crashed with a new agent that can be launched on the fly as a substitute for a failing agent (Terje and Marius 2015).

MAS are suitable for applications that require distributed and concurrent processing capabilities. They are employed in the applications in several domains such as supply chain management (Rady 2011; Zimmermann 2006; Ngan and Kanagasabai 2013), web-services (Mohamed and Makhlouf 2014; García-Sánchez et al. 2009), healthcare (Dolgui et al. 2015; Shakshuki and Reid 2015; Isern et al. 2010), e-learning (Terje and Marius 2015), etc. When a group of individual agents constitutes MAS, it is crucial to have a mechanism that can control such a group. Communication is a key for MAS to exhibit social behaviour (e.g., share information, coordinate their tasks). Individual agents in MAS interact with one another by exchanging messages using a specific Agent Communication Language (ACL). The purpose of ACL is to enable agents to convey messages to one another with meaningful statements (Vaniya et. al. 2011). Most ACLs are based on the speech-act theory. Speech acts are expressed by means of standard key words also known as communicative acts or performatives (e.g., request, inform, confirm, and propose). They are used to inform the intention of the communication from the sender to the receiver. The agent's message consists of various parameters such as sender, receiver, content language, ontology, and the actual content. Examples of well-known ACL languages are KQML (Knowledge Query and Manipulation Language) and FIPAACL (Foundations for Intelligent Physical Agents-Agents Communication Language) proposed by FIPA (The Foundation for Intelligent Physical Agents 2015). FIPA is the relevant standardisation body that promotes agent-based technology and the interoperability of its standards with other technologies.

2.6 Conclusion

Information systems research is by its nature a process of developmental enquiry, an effort to plot pathways into the future, using the tools of today and of yesterday to trawl through, mine and analyse data while ever hopeful of creating new knowledge through intellectual discovery and a process of deductive reasoning. All research is constrained by availability of resources, including time, data access and validation disciplines, and circumstances governing funding, ethics compliance and completion deadlines. Accordingly, and as much as 'completion' may be regarded as the research goal, this is never true in the context of research output value. Knowledge acquisition is a limitless endeavour.

In this book, we aim to outline the development of assistive cross-cultural communications in healthcare and employer demand intelligence systems. The former aspire to improve Australian Aboriginal type 2 diabetes healthcare communications; and the latter examines recruitment practices.

References

Berners-Lee, T.: Linked Data. Available at https://www.w3.org/DesignIssues/LinkedData (2009). Accessed 10 May 2016

Braubach, L., Alexander P., Bade, D., Krempels, K.H., Lamersdorf, W.: Deployment of distributed multi-agent systems. In: M.P. Gleizes, A. Omicini, F. Zambonelli (eds.) Engineering Societies in the Agents World V: 5th International Workshop, ESAW 2004, Toulouse, France, October 20–22, 2004. Revised Selected and Invited Papers, 261–76. Springer Berlin Heidelberg, Berlin, Heidelberg (2005)

Campbell, L.M., MacNeill, S.: The semantic web, linked and open data. JISC CETIS, The Centre for Educational Technology and Interoperability Standards (2010)

Dolgui, A., J. Sasiadek, M. Zaremba, N. Benhajji, Roy, D., Anciaux, D.: 15th IFAC Symposium on Information Control Problems in Manufacturing Patient-Centered Multi Agent System for Health Care. IFAC-PapersOnLine **48** (January), 710–14 (2015). doi:http://dx.doi.org/10.1016/j.ifacol.2015.06.166

Elamy, A.H.: Perspectives in agent-based technology. AgentLinkNews **18**, 19–22 (2005)

García-Sánchez, F., Valencia-García, R., Martínez-Béjar, R., Fernández-Breis, J.T.: An ontology, intelligent agent-based framework for the provision of semantic web services. Expert Sys. Appl. **36**, 3167–87 (2009). doi:http://dx.doi.org/10.1016/j.eswa.2008.01.037

Gruber, T.R.: Toward principles for the design of ontologies used for knowledge sharing. In: Guarino, N., Kluwer, P.R. (eds.) Academic Publishers, Deventer, The Netherlands (1993)

Heath, T., Bizer, C.: Linked Data: Evolving the Web into a global data space. Synthesis Lectures on the Semantic Web: Theory. Tech, 1–136 (2011)

Isern, D., Sánchez, D., Moreno, A.: Agents applied in health care: a review. Int. J. Med. Inform. **79**, 145–66 (2010). doi:http://dx.doi.org/10.1016/j.ijmedinf.2010.01.003

Jennings, N.R.: On agent-based software engineering. Artif. Intell. **117**, 277–296 (2000). doi:10.1016/s0004-3702(99)00107-1

Kelly, J.E., III.: Computing, Cognition and the Future of Knowing - How Humans and Machines Are Forging a New Age of Understanding. IBM White Paper (2015)

King, W.R.: Knowledge transfer. In: Encyclopedia of Knowledge Management, 2nd edn, pp. 967–76. IGI Global, Hershey, PA, USA (2010)

King, W.R., He, J.: Knowledge Sharing. In: Schwartz, D., Te'eni, D. (eds.) Encyclopedia of Knowledge Management, 2nd edn, pp. 914–23. IGI Global, Hershey, PA, USA (2010)

Kishore, R., Sharman, R., Ramesh, R.: Computational ontologies and information systems: i. foundations. Commun. Assoc. Inf. Sys. **14**, 158–183 (2004)

Mohamed, G., Makhlouf, D.: To Implement an Open-MAS Architecture for Semantic Web Services Discovery. Int. J. Agent Technol. Sys. **6**, 58–71 (2014)

Terje, K., Marius, D.: Design and Development of a multi-agent e-learning system. Int. J. Agent Technol Sys. (IJATS) **7**, 19–74 (2015). doi:10.4018/IJATS.2015040102

Ngan, L.D., Kanagasabai, R.: Semantic web service discovery: state-of-the-art and research challenges. Pers. Ubiquit. Comput. **17**, 1741–1752 (2013). doi:10.1007/s00779-012-0609-z

Pohl, C., Wuelser, G., Bebi, P., Bugmann, H., Buttler, A., Elkin, C., Grêt-Regamey, A., et al.: How to successfully publish interdisciplinary research: learning from an ecology and society special feature. Ecol. Soc. **20** (2015). doi:10.5751/es-07448-200223

Rady, H.A.: Multi-agent system for negotiation in a collaborative supply chain management. Int. J. Video Image Process. Netw. Secur. IJVIPNS-IJENS **11** (2011)

Shakshuki, E., Reid, M.: Multi-agent system applications in healthcare: current technology and future roadmap. Procedia Comput. Sci. **52**, 252–261 (2015)

Solodovnik, I.: ONTOLOGY: From philosophy to ICT and related areas. Springer-Verlag New York, Inc. (2010)

The Foundation for Intelligent Physical Agents. Available at http://www.fipa.org (2015). Accessed 10 Jan 2016

Turban, E., Sharda, R., Delen, D.: Decision Support and Business Intelligence Systems. Prentice Hall Press (2010)

Vaniya, S., Lad, B., Bhavsar, S.: A Survey on Agent Communication Languages. presented at the International Conference on Innovation, Management and Service, Singapore, September 16 (2011)

Wang, W.M., Göpfert, T., Stark, R.: Data management in collaborative interdisciplinary research projects—Conclusions from the digitalization of research in sustainable manufacturing. ISPRS Int. J. Geo-Inf. **5** (2016). doi:10.3390/ijgi5040041

Wikipedia: Financial Technology, Also Known as FinTech. Available at https://en.wikipedia.org/wiki/Financial_technology. Accessed 26 Sept 2016

Wooldridge, M., Jennings, N.R.: Intelligent agents: theory and practice. Knowl. Eng. Rev. **10**, 115–152 (1995)

Wooldridge, M.: An Introduction to Multiagent Systems. John Wiley & Sons (2009)

Ye, D., Zhang, M., Vasilakos, A.V.: A survey of self-organization mechanisms in multiagent systems. IEEE Trans. Sys. Man Cybern. Sys. 1–21 (2016). doi:10.1109/TSMC.2015.2504350

Zimmermann, R.: Agent-based supply network event management. In: Walliser, M., Brantschen, S. (eds.) Whitestein Series in Software Agent Technologies. Birkhäuser Verlag, Switzerland (2006)

Chapter 3
Ontology Engineering

3.1 Introduction

Some ontologies represent domain knowledge and organise knowledge into a specific structure e.g. hierarchy, graph, etc. Other ontologies represent formal vocabularies with well-defined axioms that allow further deductions or inferences. In whatever knowledge representation forms, ontologies shall be designed to fit a purpose. In this chapter we focus on the engineering of ontology including ontology engineering methodologies, ontology design, ontology modelling notations, and ontology editor tool.

3.2 Ontology Engineering Methodologies

There is no single consensual ontology engineering methodology. Many different ontology engineering methodologies have been proposed during the last two decades. We will consider some of them in order to illustrate the differences between them. The methodologies presented are different from each other and together cover various aspects of the ontology engineering methodologies.

There are six different ontology engineering methodologies covered and compared in this section namely:

(1) Knowledge Engineering Methodology,
(2) DOGMA Methodology,
(3) TOVE Methodology,
(4) Methontology,
(5) SENSUS Methodology, and
(6) DILIGENT Methodology.

© Springer International Publishing AG 2018

D.E. Forbes et al., *Ontology Engineering Applications in Healthcare and Workforce Management Systems*, Studies in Systems, Decision and Control 123, DOI 10.1007/978-3-319-65012-8_3

3.2.1   Knowledge Engineering Methodology

Knowledge engineering methodology (Uschold and Gruninger 1996) identifies a six-stage process for designing and maintaining ontologies.

1. Definition of the domain, purpose and scope of ontology

In this stage, description of problem domain, purpose of the ontology, and ontology scope are captured in the ontology specification document. The document includes relevant concepts, the meanings of these concepts, and their relationships.

2. Acquisition and conceptualization of the domain knowledge

The process of acquiring knowledge from a given domain requires cooperation between the ontology engineer and the domain experts. Different methods can be applied to collect and analyse the data such as domain expert interviews, survey, and text analysis of relevant documents. The informal ontology is the output of this step conceptualised domain concepts, the relationships between them, and constraints on their usage.

3. Reusing of existing ontologies

The process of developing an ontology by reusing and adapting ontological concepts from existing published ontologies is the focal point for this stage. The ultimate goal is to obtain consistency across different ontologies. The main associated processes are ontology merging and ontology alignment.

4. Formal specification of the ontology

To make them machine processable, understandable, and readable, ontologies need to be formally specified using a formal representation language. This enables machines to effectively use the ontologies.

5. Population of the ontology with individual instances

This stage focuses on analysis of ontology consistency. To define an instance of a concept, there are three steps i.e. (i) identify a concept to which the instance belongs, (ii) create instance of this concept, and (iii) determine attributes with the proper value for the instance.

6. Evaluation and documentation

As mentioned, the concepts in the ontology need to be clearly defined, coherent, and the relationships between concepts logically consistent. Consistency and completeness are the two aspects needed to evaluate the ontologies.

3.2.2   DOGMA Methodology

The DOGMA (Developing Ontology-Guided Mediations of Agents) methodology has been developed at the VUB STARLab (Vrije Universiteit Brussel Semantic Technology and Applications Research Laboratory) and is based on the principle of a double articulation (De Bo et al. 2003). DOGMA separates the specification of ontology concepts from their axioms. An ontology developed using the DOGMA double articulation approach consists of two layers: ontology base and commitment layer.

The ontology base holds the domain conceptualization i.e. ontology concepts and relationships between these concepts. The commitment layer contains (i) a set of constraints, derivation and domain rules applied to a specified subset of the ontology base (Jarrar et al. 2003), and (ii) a set of mappings between ontological elements and application elements (Deray and Verheyden 2003).

3.2.3   TOVE Methodology

The TOVE methodology (Gruninger and Fox 1995) comprises of six steps for designing ontologies.

1. Identify motivating scenarios

The development of ontologies is motivated by various scenarios which are story problems or examples that cannot be solved using the existing knowledge base, ontologies or similar techniques. Hence a new ontology or an extended ontology is required to solve the problems from motivating scenarios. A set of possible solutions to the scenario problems will be defined. The motivating scenario, together with a set of possible solutions to the scenario problems, provides an informal semantics for the concepts and relationships between those concepts. The concepts and relationships are then included in the ontology. One or more motivating scenario(s) need to be defined along with the set of possible solutions for the problems presented in the scenarios in order to design a new ontology or extending an existing ontology.

2. Formulate informal competency questions

The informal competency questions in natural language forms are used to evaluate the expressiveness of the ontology. Thus the ontology that has been expressed in a formal language needs to be able to answer these questions. The terminology, definitions and axioms are used in ontology development to represent these questions and characterize the answers to these questions.

3. Specify terminology within a formal language

There are two parts to this step i.e. (i) extraction of informal terminology and (ii) formal specification of the terminology. For extraction of informal terminology, the set of terms used within informal competency questions is extracted and serves as a basis for specification of the terminology in a formal language. For formal specification of the terminology, a formalism can be used to specify the ontology terminology. This will enable the use of axioms to express ontology definitions and constraints. If we use first order logic as a formalism to specify the ontology terminology, we firstly need to identify objects in the universe of discourse. We then need to identify unary predicates for concepts, binary predicates for attributes, and predicates for binary relations.

4. Formulate formal competency questions using formal terminology

In this step, the identified competency questions are defined formally according to the specifications.

5. Specify axioms and definitions within a formal language

A set of terms and a set of axioms in an ontology define the semantics or meaning of ontology terms. Ontology axioms define the ontology terms and specify the restrictions on their interpretation. In a case that the existing axioms are inadequate to represent and define the solutions to the competency questions in a formal language; additional axioms need to be added to the ontology. The ontology development is an iterative process here in the methodology.

6. Specify conditions characterizing ontology completeness

In the last step, the conditions need to be defined for which the solutions to the formal competency questions are complete. These conditions then serve as a basis for development of ontology completeness theorems.

3.2.4   Methontology

The METHONTOLOGY framework (Fernández-López et al. 1997) has two levels in ontology construction i.e. (i) an ontology development process and (ii) an ontology life cycle based on evolving prototypes.

1. Ontology Development Process

In this process, there are various activities needed to be carried out to construct ontologies. The activities have been identified into three categories i.e. ontology management activities (scheduling, control, and quality assurance), ontology development-oriented activities (pre-development, development, and post-development), and ontology support activities (knowledge acquisition, evaluation, integration, documentation, and configuration management).

2. Ontology Life Cycle

This is based on evolving prototypes. There are sets of phases through which the ontology develops during its life and activities performed in each phase. Ontology improvement is achieved through changes required in the evolving prototypes.

3.2.5   SENSUS Methodology

This approach is based on the assumption that if two ontologies have a common underlying structure, the knowledge can be shared. SENSUS (Swartout et al. 1997) is an ontology providing a broad coverage conceptual structure. It is composed of upper, middle and lower regions. According to the SENSUS methodology, there are five steps to be followed when building an ontology for a particular domain: (i) Identifying seed terms, (ii) Manually linking the seed terms to SENSUS, (iii) Adding paths to the root, (iv) Adding new domain terms, and (v) Adding complete subtrees.

Seed terms are considered as relevant domain specific concepts being identified and manually linked to the SENSUS ontology. Paths are to be added to the root. It could be a large number of paths in some nodes. If many nodes in a subtree are found to be relevant for the ontology, other nodes in the subtree are likely to be relevant hence the entire subtree shall be added to the ontology structure. This requires understanding of the domain.

3.2.6   DILIGENT Methodology

DILIGENT (DIstributed, Loosely-controlled and evolvInG Engineering of oNTologies) is a methodology that was developed to support domain experts in a distributed setting to engineer and evolve ontologies using a fine-grained methodological approach based on Rhetorical Structure Theory (Pinto et al. 2004). There are five main activities for DILIGENT methodology i.e. (i) building, (ii) local adaption, (iii) analysis, (iv) revision, and (v) local update.

Different stakeholders have different purposes and needs and may locate in different places for distributed ontology development. Domain experts, users, and ontology engineers firstly build an initial ontology. The ontology is made available and users can start using it. The users adapt the ontology needs locally for their own purposes. The ontology can be changed in their local environment, but the original ontology that is shared by all users may not be changed. The control board collects and analyzes change requests to the shared ontology. The board will then decide which change(s) need to be made in the next version of the shared ontology. Once a new version of the shared ontology has been released, users can locally update their own ontologies. The activities start again in iterative manner.

3.2.7 *Discussion*

In this section we compare the ontology engineering methodologies discussed above in two main aspects i.e. development and support. For the development aspect, we look into the development type and the development life cycle. We also analyse whether a methodology supports the notions of collaborative construction, ontology reusability, and ontology evolution. Table 3.1 shows a comparison of methodologies based on five features in two main aspects.

Different methodologies focus on different development models i.e. either stage, layer, step, or activity model. Some models propose an ontology life cycle which identifies the set of stages through which the ontology moves during its life. We analyse type of overall development model a methodology will follow and whether a methodology clearly recommends a life cycle or not.

Support in collaborative construction allows users, developers, evaluators, stakeholders, etc. to work on a single ontology development at the same time without a geographical location restriction. Although ontologies can be developed in isolation however community involvement in the ontology development would improve the quality of ontology. An ontology which has been developed in isolation by the domain experts who make assumptions on user requirement may quickly become obsolete and be useless to the community of users. It is then important to analyse whether a methodology supports collaborative construction or not.

Methodologies that support reusability allow ontology developers to make use of existing ontologies in order to reduce development time and effort. The adoption of ontologies bring a reusability factor (Ashraf et al. 2012) of the knowledge to the fore which is one of the core contributions of ontology use. Reused ontologies can be adopted and user in the community to produce network effects. It was also highlighted in Hepp (2007) that "ontologies exhibit positive network effects, such that their perceived utility increases with the number of people who commit to them which comes with wider usage". Ashraf et al. (2012) proposed the Ontology Usage Analysis Framework which empirically analyse the use of ontologies and ranks them based on their usage. The discussed methodologies are analysed for reusability aspect.

Ontology evolution was defined as 'the timely adaptation of ontology to the arisen changes and consistent propagation of these changes to dependent artefacts' (Stojanovic et al. 2004). The evolution is triggered by two conditions i.e. ontology domain changes and consistency management (Martins and Silva 2009). Some methodologies support ontology evolution and establish techniques to handle the changes to ontology.

Some methodologies support interoperability by interlinking with other relevant entities. Domain ontologies developed using these methodologies share the same skeleton and encourage information interoperability. The system implementing these ontologies will have a similar domain knowledge. Hence, knowledge sharing and communication will be relatively easy. It is important to analyse for ontology engineering whether the methodology supports interoperability or not.

Table 3.1 Ontology Engineering Methodologies on development and support aspects

Methodologies	Development		Support			
	Type	Life Cycle	Collaboration	Reusability	Evolution	Interoperability
Knowledge Engineering Methodology Uschold and Gruninger (1996)	Stage model	Yes	No	Yes	Yes	No
DOGMA De Bo et al. (2003)	Layer model	Yes	Not specifically mention	Not specifically mention	Yes	Yes
TOVE Gruninger and Fox (1995)	Stage model	No	No	Yes	No	No
METHONTOLOGY Fernandez et al. (1997)	Staged model	Yes	No	Yes	Yes	No
SENSUS Swartout et al. (1997)	Step model	No	Yes	Yes	Yes	Yes
DILIGENT Pinto et al. (2004)	Activity model	Yes	Yes	Yes	Yes	Yes

3.3   Ontology Design

A well-designed ontology should conform to capital questions of 'what is it about?', 'why do we need it?', and 'where do we find reusable knowledge?'. These questions constitute the problem space and the answers to the questions form a solution space. During the ontology design process, a set of criteria is important as a guidance as well as for evaluation purposes. Gruber suggests five design criteria for ontologies (Gruber 1993): Clarity, Coherence, Extendibility, Minimal Encoding Bias, and Minimal Ontological Commitment.

3.3.1   Clarity

Reasons for choosing a set of ontology concepts or classes and the intended meanings of those concepts need to be clear. There should be a restriction on the number of possible interpretations. Complete definitions of ontology concepts are preferred over partial definitions. The ontology concept definition is defined by necessary and sufficient conditions. The definitions need to be objective, documented in natural language but specified in formal axioms within the ontology. Clear definitions of ontology concepts contribute to the effectiveness of communication among agents and humans, and between agents and humans.

3.3.2   Coherence

Propositions inferred from the ontology definitions and axioms should not contradict other ontology definitions and axioms. Inferences need to be consistent with the existing definitions and axioms, and should be clear and logical.

3.3.3   Extendibility

New knowledge emerges all the time hence the new knowledge may need to be incorporated to the existing ontology. The ontology then needs to be extendable. The new ontology concepts should just be defined based on the existing vocabulary and/or ideally without the need to alter the existing ontology definitions. Extending of an ontology could result in another new ontology that contains more precise and correct definitions.

3.3.4 Minimal Encoding Bias

Conceptualizations of any domain knowledge need to be specified at a knowledge-level and not at a symbol-level. The ontology aims to represent facts. However, ontology correctness could be compromised as it is fit for purpose. The ontology correctness should not be compromised for the convenience of its notation or implementation.

3.3.5 Minimal Ontological Commitment

In the ontology, more commitments make the ontology structure more rigid and limit the number of ontology users. Ontological commitment needs to be minimal as it is sufficient to support the intended knowledge sharing activities. It may be necessary to specify an ontology which is necessary called the necessary ontology.

3.4 Logical Consistency Verification of Ontology

Ensuring an ontology is consistent is an important part of ontology development and testing. It is especially important when a shared ontology is necessary for meaningful communication. If a shared ontology is inconsistent, no reliable conclusion may be deduced. Consistency validation through reasoner for PPAC ontology includes consistency checking, concept satisfiability, classification and realization. These services are all the standard inference services traditionally provided by a reasoner, e.g. Pellet, Racerpro, etc. The differences between various reasoners were reviewed in Dentler et al. (2011).

It is important to ensure an ontology does not contain any contradictory facts in which logical consistency of the ontology is checked through a reasoner. An ontology may have concept satisfiability, i.e. a class in the ontology can have instances. In a case, if a class is unsatisfiable, then defining an instance of that class will cause the whole ontology to be inconsistent. An ontology may have a complete class hierarchy providing classification service. The class hierarchy can be used to answer queries e.g. for usability validation. The most specific class, that an instance belongs to, can be found in the ontology providing realization service. It is essential to ensure the developed ontology is consistent before consumption.

3.5 Ontology Editor Tool—Protégé

In the last decades, there has been an increase in the development of ontology editors, some of which include OntoEdit (Sure et al. 2002), Protégé (Musen 2015), OilEd (Bechhofer et al. 2001), GATE (Bontcheva et al. 2004), just to name a few.

Protégé is the most widely, commonly used ontology editor with large number of users, over three hundred thousand users at the time of writing. Many Fortune 500 companies use protégé to build their ontologies (Musen 2015).

Protégé emerged in 1987 and is still going strong. It has undergone several development phases, each of which is an improvement on the previous version with the most recent version being Protégé 5.0 at time of writing. Protégé assists developers to construct reusable ontologies and to build knowledge based systems (Musen 2015).

There are currently two platforms for Protégé i.e. a desktop system and a web-based system aka WebProtege. Protégé desktop system supports various advanced features enabling construction as well as management of ontologies. WebProtege offers distributed access over the Internet. It is Protégé client networking with Protégé server. WebProtege ontologies can be shared among distributed team members just like Google doc. This allows collaboration in ontology development and support many ontology engineering tasks. WebProtege remains the most popular web-based ontology editor that are available.

There is a vast library of Protégé plug-ins that users have developed added more features to Protégé. At the time of writing there is influx of new plug-ins in various types (e.g. reasoners, API, Import, Export, View, etc.) and topics (e.g. Visualisation, Software Engineering, Validation, NLP, Evolution, etc.).

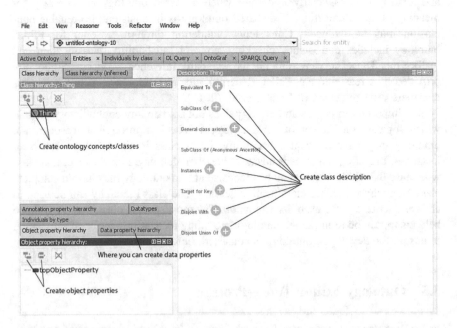

Fig. 3.1 Protégé screenshot illustrating where you can create ontology concepts/classes, class description, object properties, and data properties

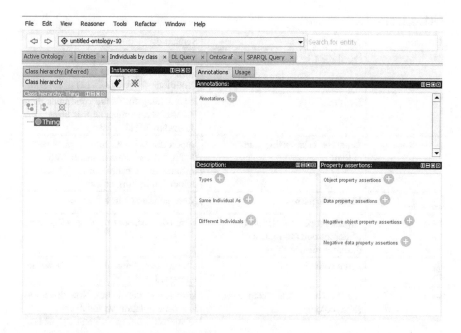

Fig. 3.2 Protégé screenshot illustrating where you can create instance(s)/individual(s) and its annotations, description, and property assertions. *Note* that screen shots are captured from the Protégé 5.0, the latest version at the time of writing

Figure 3.1 shows Protégé screenshot illustrating where you can create ontology concepts/classes, class description, object properties, and data properties. Figure 3.2 shows Protégé screenshot illustrating where you can create instance(s)/individual(s) and its annotations, description, and property assertions.

3.6   Ontology Notations

To ease understanding of the ontology model, we use OntoGraf for graphical presentation. The graphical notations are accordingly discussed in this section to facilitate the ontology modelling process. Table 3.2 shows a list of notations used in this book.

In context, class, property, and individual are written in italic style to distinguish from the text. In order to maintain consistency with names there are naming conventions for each ontology component. All class names start with a capital letter and have the remaining word(s) capitalised; and underscores are used to join words for example *Ontology_Class*. Property names or relationship names start with a lower case letter, have no spaces and have the remaining word(s) capitalised. Relationship names are prefixed with verb or adverb e.g. the words 'has', 'in', or 'related' for

Table 3.2 Modelling notations

Notation	Terminology	Semantics
●	Primitive Class	If something is a member of this class then it is necessary to fulfil the conditions (Horridge 2011)
⊜	Defined Class	If something fulfils the conditions then it must be a member of this class (Horridge 2011)
——▷——	Subclass Relationship (pink colour)	Superclass-subclass hierarchy. Note that it has the same notation with instance relationship but in different colour i.e. in pink colour
⊞ or ▶	More Subclasses	More subclasses in a hierarchy
——▷——	Object Property Relationship (different colours represent different relationships)	Link two instances or classes together
◆	Instance/Individual	Objects in the domain in which we are interested
——▷——	Instance/Individual Relationship (blue colour)	Instances of the classes. Note that it has the same notation with subclass relationship but in different colour i.e. in blue colour

example *hasRelationship*. This naming convention is used to allow for the possibility to generate more human readable expressions for descriptions. Instance or individual names start with a lower case letter and have the remaining word(s) in lower case; and underscores are used to join words for example *instance_or_individual*. In parts of the following sections, single words used in the context of query triggers are not italicised as they represent real-world human generated concept descriptions.

3.7 Conclusion

In this chapter, we introduced different ontology engineering methodologies i.e. Knowledge Engineering Methodology, DOGMA Methodology, TOVE Methodology, Methontology, SENSUS Methodology, and DILIGENT Methodology. To illustrate the diversity in ontology engineering methodologies, we discussed and compared the methodologies in developmental and supporting aspects. To make ontology development complete, design criteria and the verification process have been presented. In addition a well-known ontology editor tool named Protégé has been explained so the ontology development can be started using this modest tool.

In the following chapters, development of two ontologies and its applications will be illustrated. The integration of the two ontologies is also presented in later chapter.

References

Ashraf, J., Hussain, O.K., Hussain, F.K.: A framework for measuring ontology usage on the web. Comp J (2012)

Bechhofer, S., Horrocks, I., Goble, C., Stevens, R.: OilEd: a reason-able ontology editor for the semantic web. In: F. Baader, G. Brewka, T. Eiter (eds.) KI 2001: Advances in Artificial Intelligence: Joint German/Austrian Conference on AI Vienna, Austria, September 19–21, 2001 Proceedings, Springer Berlin Heidelberg, Berlin, Heidelberg, 396–408 2001

Bontcheva, K., Tablan, V., Maynard, D., Cunningham, H.: Evolving GATE to meet new challenges in language engineering. Nat. Lang. Eng. **10**(3–4), 349–373 (2004). doi:10.1017/s1351324904003468

De Bo, J., Spyns, P., Meersman, R.: Creating a "DOGMAtic" multilingual ontology infrastructure to support a semantic portal. In: Meersman, R., Tari, Z. (eds.) On The Move to Meaningful Internet Systems 2003: OTM 2003 Workshops: OTM Confederated International Workshops, HCI-SWWA, IPW, JTRES,WORM, WMS, and WRSM 2003, Catania, Sicily, Italy, November 3–7, 2003. Proceedings, Springer Berlin Heidelberg, Berlin, Heidelberg, pp. 253–266 (2003)

Dentler, K., Cornet, R., ten Teije, A., de Keizer, N.: Comparison of reasoners for large ontologies in the OWL 2 EL profile. Semant. web **2**(2), 71–87 (2011). doi:10.3233/sw-2011-0034

Deray, T., Verheyden, P.: Towards a semantic integration of medical relational databases by using ontologies: a case study. In: Meersman, R., Tari, Z. (eds.) On The Move to Meaningful Internet Systems 2003: OTM 2003 Workshops: OTM Confederated International Workshops, HCI-SWWA, IPW, JTRES,WORM, WMS, and WRSM 2003, Catania, Sicily, Italy, November 3–7, 2003. Proceedings, Springer Berlin Heidelberg, Berlin, Heidelberg, pp. 137–150 (2003)

Fernández-López, M., Gómez-Pérez, A., Juristo, N.: Methontology: from ontological art towards ontological engineering. AAAI-97 Spring Symposium Series, Stanford University, EEUU (1997)

Gruber, T.R.: Toward principles for the design of ontologies used for knowledge sharing. In: International Workshop on Formal Ontology in Conceptual Analysis and Knowledge Representation, Padova, Italy (1993)

Gruninger, M., Fox, M.: Methodology for the design and evaluation of ontologies. In: IJCAI'95, Workshop on Basic Ontological Issues in Knowledge Sharing, 13 Apr 1995

Hepp, M.: Possible ontologies: how reality constrains the development of relevant ontologies. Internet Comput **11**(1), 90–96 (2007)

Martins, H., Silva, N.: A User-driven and a Semantic-based Ontology Mapping Evolution Approach. ICEIS (2009)

Musen, M.A.: The protege project: a look back and a look forward. AI Matters **1**(4), 4–12 (2015). doi:10.1145/2757001.2757003

Mustafa, J., Demey, J., Meersman, R.: On using conceptual data modeling for ontology engineering. In: S. Spaccapietra, S. March, K. Aberer (eds.) Journal on Data Semantics I, Springer Berlin Heidelberg, Berlin, Heidelberg, 185–207 (2003)

Pinto, H.S., Steffen, S., Tempich, C.: DILIGENT: Towards a Fine-grained Methodology for Distributed, Loosely-controlled and Evolving Engineering of oNTologies. ECAI (2004)

Stojanovic, N., Studer, R., Stojanovic, L.: An Approach for Step-By-Step Query Refinement in the Ontology-Based Information Retrieval. Web Intelligence, 2004. WI 2004. In: Proceedings. IEEE/WIC/ACM International Conference on, 20–24 Sept 2004

Sure, Y., Erdmann, M., Angele, J., Staab, S., Studer, R., Wenke, D.: OntoEdit: Collaborative Ontology Development for the Semantic Web. In: Horrocks, I. I., Hendler, J. (eds.) The Semantic Web—ISWC 2002: First International Semantic Web Conference Sardinia, Italy, June 9–12, 2002 Proceedings, Springer Berlin Heidelberg, Berlin, Heidelberg, pp. 221–235 (2002)

Swartout, B., Patil, R., Knight, K., Russ, T.: Toward Distributed Use of Large-Scale Ontologies. In: Ontological Engineering, AAAI-97 Spring Symposium Series (1997)

Uschold, M., Gruninger, M.: Ontologies: principles, methods and applications. Know. Eng. Rev. **11**(2) (1996)

Chapter 4
Patient Practitioner Assistive Communications Ontology

4.1 Introduction

In the previous chapter, ontology engineering including different methodologies, design criteria, verification process, and editor tool are presented. That gives a general understanding of ontology development. In this chapter, we present specifically the development of PPAC ontology. It provides briefly all PPAC ontology classes and subclasses, properties, and constraints. The fine detailed development of the PPAC ontology can be found in Forbes (2013). The PPAC ontology is a main component of healthcare communication systems which will be covered in the next chapter.

4.2 Overview of PPAC Ontology

PPAC ontology represents Type II diabetes terminologies together with Aboriginal English (AE) home talk. The objective is to help General Practitioners (GPs) and Aboriginal patients storing and communicating general Type II diabetes knowledge and patient-related information efficiently. The PPAC ontology supports the need of Aboriginal Type II diabetes healthcare process to transmit, reuse and share patient data.

The practitioner objective is as follows. First is to identify T2DM standard concept equivalents of patient AE words, phrases or expressions. Second is to identify AE words, phrases or expressions suited to the consultation context. Third is to semantically identify relevant AE properties.

The patient-oriented objective is as follows. First is to guide the practitioner towards cultural competence. Second is to find AE concept equivalents of Type II diabetes words, phrases or expressions. Third is to guide the practitioner towards links with relevant AE PPAC concepts.

© Springer International Publishing AG 2018
D.E. Forbes et al., *Ontology Engineering Applications in Healthcare
and Workforce Management Systems*, Studies in Systems,
Decision and Control 123, DOI 10.1007/978-3-319-65012-8_4

The PPAC ontology has been developed for Type II Diabetes in which a standardised vocabulary drawn from Type II diabetes management guidelines is captured along with AE home talk. The two domain knowledge contributions are captured, i.e. Type II diabetes concepts which classify all concepts related to Type II diabetes and AE home talk concepts which classify all concepts used in Aboriginal communications. These two domain knowledge contributions are linked together through ontology relations and constraints. Type II diabetes and AE concepts are self-standing and independent domains. The refining and dependent concepts are value types and values which partition conceptual spaces. The dependent concepts are the concepts of

- complication risk (either high, moderate, or low),
- medication advice (either adherence or interaction),
- observation (either extrinsic or intrinsic), and
- testing type (clinical examination, point of care tests, and/or self-management).

Figure 4.1 illustrates the refining concepts.

PPAC ontology has been developed in OWL using Protégé 5.0. It contains 787 logical axioms, 221 classes, 22 object properties, 7 data properties and 130 instances. The PPAC ontology does not contain any contradictory facts in which logical consistency of the ontology is checked through Pellet and Racerpro. The PPAC ontology has also concept satisfiability, i.e. a class in PPAC ontology can have instances. If a class is unsatisfiable, then defining an instance of that class will cause the whole ontology to be inconsistent. The PPAC ontology has a complete class hierarchy (classification service). The class hierarchy can be used to answer queries, usability validation. The most specific class, that an instance belongs to, can be found in the PPAC ontology (realization service). From our experiment the PPAC ontology is consistent and ready for consumption.

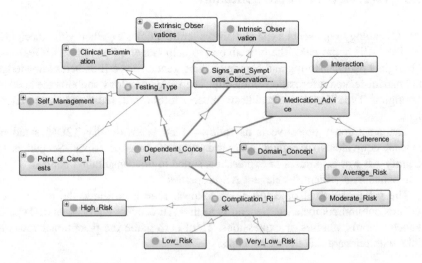

Fig. 4.1 Refining concepts

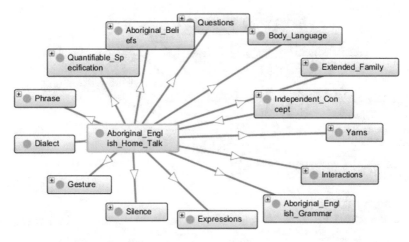

Fig. 4.2 Subclasses of the main class *Aboriginal_English_Home_Talk*

4.3   Aboriginal English Home Talk Ontology Classes

Aboriginal English Home Talk concepts drawn from the Aboriginal English education research, focus group, and mentor contact sources of knowledge are conceptualised into ontology classes which classify Aboriginal communications.
Figure 4.2 shows the main class *Aboriginal_English_Home_Talk* with its subclasses. Figures 4.3 and 4.4 show the other subclasses. The classes are organised
into a super class-subclass hierarchy, where subclasses are subsumed into their
respective super classes. As an example, those yarns, Aboriginal beliefs, gesture,
etc. are Aboriginal communication as in English home talk.

4.4   Type 2 Diabetes Ontology Classes

Type 2 Diabetes concepts drawn from published RACGP Guidelines are conceptualised into ontology classes which are structured to facilitate the mapping of
clinical language with the Aboriginal English home talk through class relationships
and constraints. Figure 4.5 shows the main class *Type_2_Diabetes_Concepts* with
its subclasses. Figures 4.6 and 4.7 show the other subclasses.

4.5   Object and Data Properties

For the process of building a valid ontology, the representation of relationships is
important. These are represented through object and data properties. The object
properties represent relationships between two classes or two individuals while the

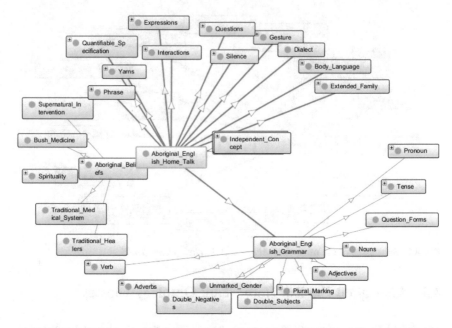

Fig. 4.3 Subclasses of class *Aboriginal_Beliefs* and subclasses of class *Aboriginal_English_Grammar*

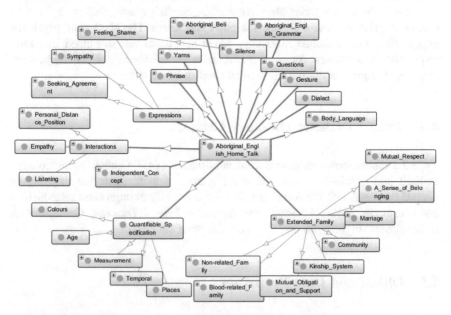

Fig. 4.4 Subclasses of class *Interaction*; subclasses of class *Expression*; subclasses of class *Extended_Family*; subclasses of class *Quantifiable_Specification*

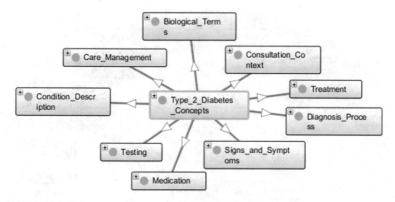

Fig. 4.5 Subclasses of the main class *Type_2_Diabetes_Concepts*

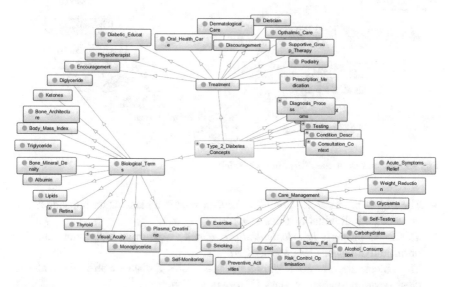

Fig. 4.6 Subclasses of class *Biological_Terms*; subclasses of class *Treatment*; subclasses of class *Care_Management*

data properties describe relationships between a class or an individual and data values such as an Extensible Markup Language (XML) Schema Datatype or RDF literal, which accommodates class values such as strings and integers using a lexical format.

There are three types of object property in PPAC ontology i.e. *refiningProperty*, *relatedAboriginalEnglishHomeTalk*, and *relatedType2DiabetesConcepts* as shown in Fig. 4.8.

The object property *refiningProperty* has four sub properties and the following shows its relationships:

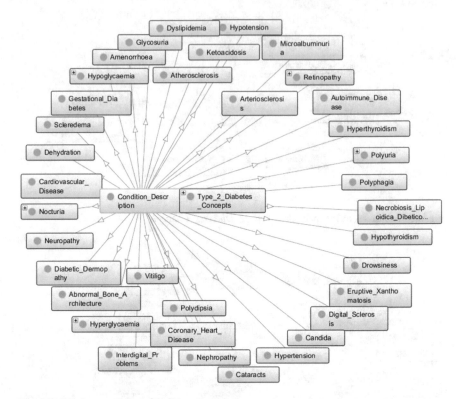

Fig. 4.7 Subclasses of class *Condition_Description*

- The object property *hasComplicationRisk* relates a class or an individual with class or an individual of class *Complication_Risk*.
- The object property *hasMedicalAdvice* relates a class or an individual with class or an individual of class *Medical_Advice*.
- The object property *hasObservationType* relates a class or an individual with class or an individual of class *Observation_Type*.
- The object property *hasTestingType* relates a class or an individual with class or an individual of class *Testing_Type*.

The object property *relatedAboriginalEnglishHomeTalk* has five sub properties and the following shows its relationships:

- The object property *hasBeliefs* relates a class or an individual with class or an individual of class *Beliefs*.
- The object property *hasExpressivity* relates a class or an individual with class or an individual of class *Expressivity*.
- The object property *hasExtendedFamily* relates a class or an individual with class or an individual of class *Extended_Family*.

Fig. 4.8 Object properties
and its sub object properties
in PPAC ontology

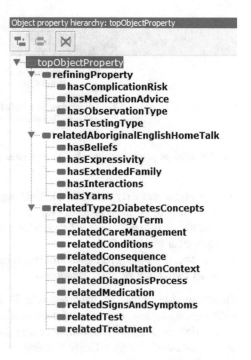

- The object property *hasInteractions* relates a class or an individual with class or an individual of class *Interactions*.
- The object property *hasYarns* relates a class or an individual with class or an individual of class *Yarns*.

The object property *relatedType2DiabetesConcepts* has ten sub properties and the following shows its relationships:

- The object property *relatedBiologyTerm* relates a class or an individual with class or an individual of class *Biology_Term*.
- The object property *relatedCareManagement* relates a class or an individual with class or an individual of class *Care_Management*.
- The object property *relatedConditions* relates a class or an individual with class or an individual of class *Conditions*.
- The object property *relatedConsequence* relates a class or an individual with class or an individual of class *Consequence*.
- The object property *relatedConsultationContext* relates a class or an individual with class or an individual of class *Consultation_Context*.
- The object property *relatedDiagnosisProcess* relates a class or an individual with class or an individual of class *Diagnosis_Process*.
- The object property *relatedMedication* relates a class or an individual with class or an individual of class *Medication*.

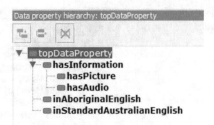

Fig. 4.9 Data properties and its sub data properties in PPAC ontology

- The object property *relatedSignsAndSymptoms* relates a class or an individual with class or an individual of class *Signs_And_Symptoms.*
- The object property *relatedTest* relates a class or an individual with class or an individual of class *Test.*
- The object property *relatedTreatment* relates a class or an individual with class or an individual of class *Treatment.*

There are three types of data property in PPAC ontology i.e. *hasInformation*, in*AboriginalEnglish*, and *inStandardAustralianEnglish* as shown in Fig. 4.9.

The data properties *hasInformation and its sub properties*, *inAboriginalEnglish*, and *inStandardAustralianEnglish* relate a class or an individual with string. Figure 4.10 shows the examples of the usage:

- Data property *hasAudio* relates individual *big* with XML Schema Datatype of string 'c:\\Audio\\big'. Instance *big* has relation *hasAudio* with a string which is showed where its audio locates. This infers to an audio file recording of an aboriginal English voice being heard to say 'big' in elongated version to represent AE mode of measurement emphasis.
- Data property *inAboriginalEnglish* relates individual *alcohol* with XML Schema Datatype of string 'good stuff'. Instance *alcohol* has relation *inAboriginal English* with a string 'good stuff'. This infers that alcohol in Standard English refer to good stuff in Aboriginal English.

> ◆ big hasAudio "c:\\Audio\\big"^^xsd:string
>
> ◆ alcohol inAboriginalEnglish "good stuff"^^xsd:string
>
> ◆ uncle inStandardAustralianEnglish "uncle"^^xsd:string
> ◆ uncle inStandardAustralianEnglish "nephew"^^xsd:string

Fig. 4.10 Example of data property usage

- Data property *inStandardAustralianEnglish* relates individual *uncle* with XML Schema Datatype of string 'uncle' and 'nephew'. Instance *uncle* has relation *inStandardAustralianEnglish* with a string 'uncle' and a string 'nephew'. This infers that uncle in Aboriginal English can refer to uncle as well as nephew in Standard English.

4.6   Instance Populations

Ontology instances or individuals represent concrete information specified as an instance of one or several ontology classes. Ontology classes represent the concepts defined as the specification of a group of instances that belong together because they share some properties. Figure 4.11 shows number of instances in each class.

Figure 4.12 shows individual of class *Extended_Family* and its subclasses. As can be seen from the figure, brother and grandchildren are not only blood related family but can also be non-related family. Likewise female are non-related family but also can be blood-related family too. This reflects Aboriginal culture and how we conceptualise it in PPAC ontology. From this reference it shows that the notions of extended family and community as family in Aboriginal communities encompass the idea that children are not just the concern of the biological parents, but of the entire community. The raising, care, education and discipline of children are the responsibility of everyone—male, female, young and old. This reflects community as family.

4.7   Case Study

In this section we provide a case scenario to project briefly the use of PPAC ontology in circumstances where the patient-practitioner relationship and consultation are confronted with communications difficulties. Further detailed case studies and its source can also be found in Forbes and Wongthongtham (2016), Forbes et al. (2013).

A 28 year old Nyungar male 'Vincent' is in the care of a fifty-eight year old close community friend 'Ted' who while not blood related he refers to as 'uncle'. Both have been living for an unknown period of time in bushland in and around the south west of Australia. Together they attend a country health clinic by appointment, and initially the older man enters the doctor's office alone. He is surprised to discover that the GP, Dr. Rose, is a white European-born female. He tells her that he wants a male doctor to examine his 'huncle' but that the patient is refusing to come in from the waiting area due to embarrassment. The only person in the waiting room at that time she notes is Vincent who is visibly unwell and suffering dizziness but could not possibly be (in her view) Ted's uncle.

Fig. 4.11 Number of individuals for each class in PPAC ontology

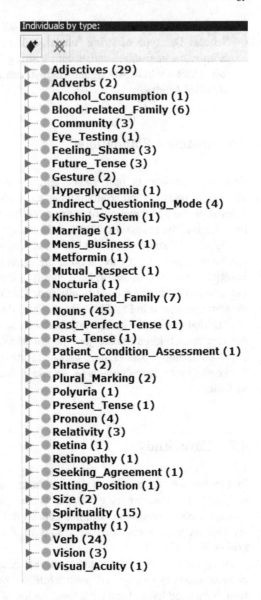

Individuals by type:

- Adjectives (29)
- Adverbs (2)
- Alcohol_Consumption (1)
- Blood-related_Family (6)
- Community (3)
- Eye_Testing (1)
- Feeling_Shame (3)
- Future_Tense (3)
- Gesture (2)
- Hyperglycaemia (1)
- Indirect_Questioning_Mode (4)
- Kinship_System (1)
- Marriage (1)
- Mens_Business (1)
- Metformin (1)
- Mutual_Respect (1)
- Nocturia (1)
- Non-related_Family (7)
- Nouns (45)
- Past_Perfect_Tense (1)
- Past_Tense (1)
- Patient_Condition_Assessment (1)
- Phrase (2)
- Plural_Marking (2)
- Polyuria (1)
- Present_Tense (1)
- Pronoun (4)
- Relativity (3)
- Retina (1)
- Retinopathy (1)
- Seeking_Agreement (1)
- Sitting_Position (1)
- Size (2)
- Spirituality (15)
- Sympathy (1)
- Verb (24)
- Vision (3)
- Visual_Acuity (1)

The doctor is somewhat confused but realises there is a communications barrier. Her training should enable her to consider how to resolve this quandary. The option of querying an ontology supported PPAC system would help her to navigate through a search of consultation context subclasses and attributes to learn more specifically how she might handle this situation.

From the above scenario Dr. Rose could query search for the word 'huncle' to find its possible meaning. The word 'huncle' in AE can be taken to mean 'uncle'

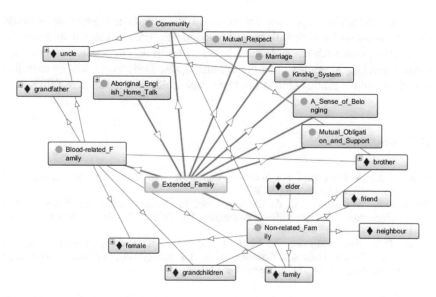

Fig. 4.12 Individual of class *Extended_Family* and its subclasses

and also to mean 'nephew' in Standard English. This refers to bi-directionality in the uncle and nephew relationship. As can be seen in Fig. 4.12, individual uncle is also an individual of classes *Blood-related_Family*, *Community*, *Kinship_System*, *Marriage*, and *Mutual_Respect*.

Dr. Rose can also navigate through the concepts. Looking into class *Consultation_Context* which has class *Accompanied_Patient* as subclass, there is relation called *hasExtendedFamily* which links to class *Extended_Family*. With all these references, it then makes sense to infer that Vincent, accompanied by Ted, although being called his uncle may not be his blood related uncle. Hence from these references, Dr. Rose will be able to assume that the Aboriginal patient and his carer are part of a community that would treat each as 'uncle' of the other.

Another term that can cause confusion like uncle is the term 'grannies' which is commonly used to refer to Aboriginal 'grandchildren'. It presents that grannies in AE can be taken to mean grandchildren in SE and it is an individual of class *Blood-related_Family*.

4.8 Conclusion

The development of PPAC ontology has been reported providing PPAC ontology classes and its subclasses, properties, constraints, and individuals. The case study has shown the use of PPAC ontology in communication difficulty circumstances. The PPAC ontology is a main component of healthcare communication systems which is a dynamic support system to elevate the pragmatic experience of health care consultations for both patients and practitioners. The challenge is to enrich the information source schema and semantic quality of the data to populate and map the merged ontology systems so that the eventual applications model will be attractive to and its use ubiquitous among the major stakeholders in health care PPIEs.

References

Forbes, D.E.: A Framework For Assistive Communications Technology In Cross-Cultural Healthcare. Curtin University (2013)

Forbes, D.E., Wongthongtham, P.: Ontology based intercultural patient practitioner assistive communications from qualitative gap analysis. Inf. Techno. People **29**, 280–317 (2016). doi:10.1108/ITP-08-2014-0166

Forbes, D.E., Wongthongtham, P., Singh, J., Thompson, S.: Ontology supported assistive communications in healthcare. Commun. Assoc. Inf. Sys. (CAIS). http://aisel.aisnet.org/cgi/viewcontent.cgi?article=3737&context=cais (2013)

Chapter 5
Cross-Cultural Healthcare Communication System

5.1 Introduction

In the previous chapter, how PPAC ontology is developed is presented. It shows all concepts, properties, and instances along with some case studies to understand the ontology use. In this chapter, we present healthcare communications systems in which the PPAC ontology and knowledge base are placed as main components. It presents how data and knowledge are assimilated in and dissimilated from the PPAC ontology. Ultimately the systems will continuously grow with expansion of knowledge.

5.2 System Architecture

The system architecture of ontology based application for healthcare communication systems as shown in Fig. 5.1 consists of two phases namely knowledge assimilation and knowledge dissimilation. The knowledge assimilation phase is for capturing and representing the aboriginal healthcare domain knowledge in a formal conceptual model. The knowledge dissimilation phase exposes the captured domain knowledge and its knowledge base to the different type of users and applications. Both phases are discussed in detail in the following subsections.

5.2.1 Knowledge Assimilation

Knowledge assimilation is aimed to represent, capture, integrate, and refine the aboriginal healthcare knowledge. Schwotzer and Berlin (2008) consider knowledge assimilation as a process whereby new knowledge is captured and incorporated into

© Springer International Publishing AG 2018
D.E. Forbes et al., *Ontology Engineering Applications in Healthcare and Workforce Management Systems*, Studies in Systems, Decision and Control 123, DOI 10.1007/978-3-319-65012-8_5

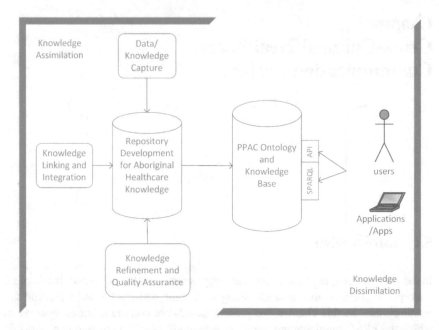

Fig. 5.1 System architecture of ontology based application for healthcare communication systems

the existing knowledge base. The knowledge is formalised in a computational and machine understandable model that is accessible to different type of applications. The captured knowledge specific to type 2 diabetes and aboriginal English home/health talk is conceptually represented in PPAC ontology which is presented in the previous chapter.

It is necessary for the concepts represented in the PPAC ontology to be aligned with other similar ontologies for increased information interoperability. For the alignment, ontology mapping techniques are used to create meaningful and context aware relationships between different terms referring to the similar concepts. Before enabling application or services to make use of the knowledge represented in the PPAC ontology and its knowledge base, the captured data should be evaluated and verified by the domain experts. This means that the captured knowledge and its mapping with different vocabularies must imply a quality assurance process to ensure the production of quality information. This quality assurance process assists in generating the commercial grade knowledge base that is exposed to the different type of users and applications.

5.2.2   *Knowledge Dissimilation*

Knowledge dissimilation is aimed to dissimilate the healthcare knowledge to different type of applications and users. To cater the diverse type of applications and user needs, the knowledge base must be represented and structured in such a way that it is capable of providing granular access to the information. Since there could be numerous applicable circumstances that will benefit from the PPAC ontology and its knowledge base, a dissimilation platform offers users and application access to information via API, querying, and/or recommendation engine for scalability and interoperability. For example, information search and retrieval can be done through querying the PPAC ontology.

5.3   System Components

Based on the system architecture shown, there are different components involved in the implementation of such systems. The system components consist of Data and Knowledge Capture, Knowledge Linking and Integration, Knowledge Refinement and Quality Assurance, and Knowledge Exposure.

5.3.1   Data and Knowledge Capture

Data capturing process is aimed to capture the raw data that comprehensively represents the domain knowledge that is being used in day-to-day discourse and social interactions. All possible raw data is captured and stored through an application namely Mobile Knowledge Capturing Application (MokCa). The captured data is subsequently used to represent the information in a more formal structure, making it understandable and process-able by different type of users including human and machines in a form of software agent for example.

MokCa is capable of recording audio and video and aimed to facilitate the fieldworker or healthcare professional by providing them with an easy-to-use application to capture the data anytime anywhere when it is available. MokCa enables users to record the local knowledge about the different healthcare related vocabularies being used within regional communities and link it with similar terminologies being used in other controlled vocabularies. MokCa has four main components namely (i) Concept Hierarchy, (ii) Specific Concepts, (iii) Annotation, and (iv) Capturing.

In the concept hierarchy component, it displays the main categories of the conceptual knowledge captured in the PPAC ontology i.e. those main concepts or super classes. Users are allowed to retrieve the specific concepts that describe the entities and domain knowledge more specifically in the specific concepts component. In the annotation component, it displays the additional information about the concepts or entities. There are different world knowledge sources which will be considered for providing the supporting information such as Auer et al. (2007), Belleau et al. (2008), and Momtchev (2009). These sources maintain a rich set of Semantic Web data that not only describes use of healthcare terminologies but also interlined with other semantic repositories. In the capturing component, it allows users to enter the local terms referring to the formal term being used in the healthcare profession lexicon. Recording audio or video is also available that help contextualize the captured information. Integration with other standard controlled vocabularies enable alignment with local knowledge with standard terminologies. The integration mechanism is discussed in the next section.

5.3.2   Knowledge Linking and Integration

Knowledge linking and Integration is designed to align the PPAC Ontology with other ontologies and controlled vocabularies to achieve information interoperability. As discussed by Noy (2009), ontology alignment is the process of determining correspondences between concepts, the outcome of which is an alignment. Generally speaking, ontology alignment tools and techniques are used to find classes of data that are semantically equivalent or similar. It can be regarded as synonyms but also may be referred to as examples of near-synonymy, depending on surrounding context. In the alignment, concepts are not necessarily logically identical however there are three possible dimensions of similarities according to Euzenat and Shvaiko (2007) i.e. syntactic, external, and semantic. There are a number of tools and frameworks that have been developed for aligning ontologies. These can be either used or extended for the specific alignment requirements. Silk framework is a tool for discovering relationships between data items within different ontologies and Linked Data sources (Bizer et al. 2009). The advantage of using Silk is that its server-side service provides a REST interface that handles an incoming data stream of newly discovered entities, while keeping track of known entities which then enables us to perform alignment with multiple knowledge bases or repositories.

The largest repository of Biomedical related ontologies is the Open Biological and Biomedical Ontologies also known as OBO Foundry (Smith et al. 2007). This repository provides numerous ontologies describing the healthcare and biomedical domain, however it lacks coverage of most of the healthcare services-related ontologies. For the longer term alignment in the PPAC ontology and its knowledge base, ICD-10 (2010) and SNOMED-CT (2016), BioPortal (NCBO's ontology repository) (Noy 2009), Ontology Lookup Service (OLS) (Côté et al. 2006) are considered. They are sophisticated systems based on medical knowledge designed to serve the professional health care domain.

5.3.3   Refinement and Quality Assurance

It is very important that the data and knowledge stored in the knowledge base is maintained at a high quality standard and integrity for it to remain useful. To ensure the high quality of the data, it requires a hybrid mechanism to verify and validate the captured data before committing it to the knowledge base. The proposed approach is based on two workspaces i.e. development and production. All the queries will be answered from the production system. Ongoing knowledge capturing and verification transactions however will be managed through the development knowledge base.

5.3.4 Knowledge Exposure

The knowledge base is essentially a semantic repository based on a graph model. It stores the information in the form of RDF statements which are essentially tuples comprising of subject, predicate and object known as resources. In the Semantic Web resources are defined using Universal Resource Identifiers (URIs) which are then used to describe the resources and interlink with other resources. The Virtuoso triple store is used to store the RDF triples, PPAC ontology, schemas. The open source edition of Virtuoso namely OpenLink Virtuoso is utilised.

There are a number of ways to expose the knowledge base. A SPARQL endpoint enables any consuming application to pose queries to the semantic repository which is in RDF triple store. In certain cases, where the consuming application is not SPARQL aware, Web API can be implemented as a REpresentational State Transfer (REST) based service (Szepielak 2008).

5.4 Applications for Cross-Cultural Healthcare Communications System

This section demonstrates how the healthcare communication systems provide a solution to a practical use case scenario. Figure 5.2 shows solution view in which the data collected, processed, and transmitted by through and from healthcare communication systems. The systems is part of the interactive communication processes. The context relevance and cross cultural communications efficacy of patient health information are facilitated by the PPAC ontology situated in the healthcare communication systems. Use case scenarios are described in following sub sections.

5.4.1 Patient Scenario

A patient in the remote community is suffering Type 2 Diabetes and plans to see a doctor in a week's time. He records and captures all the signs and symptoms that

Fig. 5.2 Solution view for healthcare communication systems

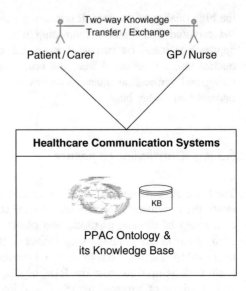

are causing concerns. The patient uses the application that is developed based on the PPAC ontology and its knowledge base to record all the events when and where they happen. All the complexity, such as the recognition of local terminology, the categorization of information, and tagging of artifacts such as images, audio files, videos with relevant medical terminologies, is hidden from the user as those are being encapsulated by the PPAC ontology and its knowledge base.

Patient assistive application enables patients to record the signs and symptoms they are or have been recently. The system encourages contemporaneous notations and thoroughness in this patient descriptions data entry/selection process. An ontology and knowledge base resource drop down menu for commonly recognized 'typical' T2DM and general Signs and Symptoms reflecting well-being perceptions will ease the stress of this exercise. From the user experience perspective, the application is designed to keep in view the target audience expertise level and to avoid unnecessary complexity. However, the application is able to perform the complex operations that interlink, map and translate the different terminologies to the user language setting and hidden from the user.

A fictional example is given to expand the explanation. The words (starting with signs and symptoms as a category) are likely to be recognized from a voice recording but will be found through the choice of a pictorial icon and a text reference. As an example, the text key words might be 'Fingers', 'Foot' or 'Hand'. All are instances of the ontology class *Signs_and_Symptoms*. This may also correlate with another instance i.e. Feeling. The patient as a diagnosed type 2 diabetic wants to confirm and record the fact that physical sensations he/she is experiencing are in need of attention and may have implications for diabetes complications.

Suffering occasional tingling feelings in his/her extremities, the patient goes to selection that includes the Aboriginal English words in textual and audio form, "Buzzing" and/or "Flashies". These terms are mapped with the Type_2_Diabetes_ Concepts clinical terminology ontology class *Condition_Description*, subclass Neuropathy. Eventually the annotations for this concept will offer Aboriginal English voice and text explanations to help the patient understand the context and possible implications of the signs and symptoms known as "Buzzing" and "Flashies". Ultimately mappings will provide the option to find self-management advice under the ontology class *Care_Management*. The ability of knowledge integration and mapping among Aboriginal English and standard healthcare terminologies opens up a dynamic new level of healthcare services for better and healthy life in remote areas.

5.4.2 GP Scenario

The GP or paramedical staff can access the information pertaining to the symptoms that are causing concerns to the patient. The information is enriched with semantically knowledge base. GP assistive application integrates the information from different sources to provide comprehensive and contextualized information to the healthcare professional. The availability of integrated information helps doctors and paramedical staff in better decision making by bridging the language gap through the use of services provided by the PPAC ontology and its knowledge base.

The ability of the healthcare communication systems to semantically annotate and describe the user intended and requested information in a machine process-able format helps in addressing several problems faced by a health professional working in or using telehealth systems to connect with patients in remote areas. This includes but is not limited to:

- Based on the user's recorded information, annotation using different labels according to the intended individual user's natural language and expertise level,
- Contextualization of the information by linking it with relevant information,
- Tagging the information for searching and clustering,
- Relating the current medical situation to the existing electronic health record,
- Integrating the medical record with hospital and clinical management systems,
- Assisting and educating healthcare workers working in remote location about the regional languages, culture and norms. This would be a perennial process aimed at building high levels of cultural competence.

Applications are developed using the APIs which allows exposure of the PPAC ontology and its knowledge base to retrieve the healthcare related knowledge.

5.5 Conclusion

We presented in this chapter healthcare communications systems in which the PPAC ontology and its knowledge base being placed as main components. The data and knowledge are assimilated in and dissimilated from the PPAC ontology making the systems continuingly grow with expansion of knowledge.

References

Auer, S., Bizer, C., Kobilarov, G., Lehmann, J., Cyganiak, R., Ives, Z.: DBpedia: a nucleus for a web of open data. In: K. Aberer, K.S. Choi, N. Noy, D. Allemang, K.I. Lee, L. Nixon, J. Golbeck, P. Mika, D. Maynard, R. Mizoguchi, G. Schreiber, P. Cudré-Mauroux (eds.) The Semantic Web: 6th International Semantic Web Conference, 2nd Asian Semantic Web Conference, ISWC 2007 + ASWC 2007, Busan, Korea, November 11–15, 2007. Proceedings, Springer Berlin Heidelberg, Berlin, Heidelberg, 722–735 (2007)

Belleau, F., Tourigny, N., Good, B., Morissette, J.: Bio2RDF: A semantic web atlas of post genomic knowledge about human and mouse. In: A. Bairoch, S. Cohen-Boulakia, C. Froidevaux (eds.) Data Integration in the Life Sciences: 5th International Workshop, DILS 2008, Evry, France, June 25–27, 2008. Proceedings, Berlin, Heidelberg: Springer Berlin Heidelberg, 153–160 (2008)

Bizer, C., Volz, J., Kobilarov, G., Gaedke, M.: Silk-A Link Discovery Framework for the Web of Data. In: 18th International World Wide Web Conference, April (2009)

Côté, R.G., Jones, P., Apweiler, R., Hermjakob, H.: The ontology lookup service, a lightweight cross-platform tool for controlled vocabulary queries. BMC Bioinformatics 7(1), 1–7 (2006). doi:10.1186/1471-2105-7-97

Euzenat, J., Shvaiko, P.: Ontology Matching. Springer-Verlag, New York, Inc (2007)

ICD-10 International Statistical Classification of Diseases and Related Health Problems. World Health Organisation (WHO). Available at http://apps.who.int/classifications/icd10/browse/2010/en (2010). Accessed 9 Jun 2015

Momtchev, V., Peychev, D., Primov, T., Georgiev, G.: Expanding the Pathway and Interaction Knowledge in Linked Life Data. International Semantic Web Challenge, Washington DC (2009)

Noy, N.F., Shah, N.H., Whetzel, P.L., Dai, B., Dorf, M., Griffith, N., Jonquet, C., Rubin, D.L., Storey, M.-A., Chute, C.G., Musen, M.A.: BioPortal: ontologies and integrated data resources at the click of a mouse. Nucl. Acids Res. (2009)

Schwotzer, T., Berlin, F.H.T.W.: Building context aware P2P systems with the shark framework. In: Fourth International Conference on Topic Maps Research and Applications, Leipzig, Germany (2008)

Smith, B., Ashburner, M., Rosse, C., Bard, J., Bug, W., Ceusters, W., Goldberg, L.J., Eilbeck, K., Ireland, A., Mungall, C.J., Leontis, N., Rocca-Serra, P., Ruttenberg, A., Sansone, S.A., Scheuermann, R.H., Shah, N., Whetzel, P.L., Lewis, S.: The OBO foundry: coordinated evolution of ontologies to support biomedical data integration. Nat. Biotechnol. 25(11), 1251–1255 (2007)

Systematized Nomenclature of Medicine—Clinical Terms SNOMED CT. International Health Terminology Standards Development Organisation (IHTSDO). Available at http://www.ihtsdo.org/snomed-ct/ (2016). Accessed 9 Nov 2016

Szepielak, D.: REST-based service oriented architecture for dynamically integrated information systems. In: PhD Symposium at ICSOC. 6, (2008)

Chapter 6
Employer Demand Ontology

6.1 Introduction

While in the previous two chapters the area of healthcare is focused, in this chapter and the next chapter workforce management area is emphasised. We firstly present development of Employer Demand Ontology (EDO) in this chapter. We then present an ontology-based Application for employer demand identification which has EDO as a key component in the next chapter. The fine detailed development of the EDO can be found in Smalberger (2013).

6.2 Overview of Employer Demand Ontology

EDO represents a shared understanding of the employer demand domain knowledge enabling efficient and intelligent management of all its existing information sources across the domain. The EDO conceptualises all the concepts relating to any occupation in Australia and it is divided into two parts. The first part represents all the concepts found in job advertisements that are relevant to determining employer demand at any given point in time. It is a high level nonspecific occupation type for general concepts that are applicable to all occupation types. The second part consists of all the types of occupations found in Australia. It is a detailed occupation specific relevant to each separate occupation as defined under the Australian and New Zealand Standard Classification of Occupations (ANZSCO). Separating the ED Ontology into two parts allows easy comparisons to be made between types of occupational dataset outputs for each period.

The EDO instance population happens through collecting job advertisements from the job board SEEK (www.seek.com.au). The specific occupations, that the data will be collected for, will be for the sixteen Nursing and Midwifery occupations from the ANZSCO. The geographical area that will be covered will be that of

© Springer International Publishing AG 2018
D.E. Forbes et al., *Ontology Engineering Applications in Healthcare and Workforce Management Systems*, Studies in Systems, Decision and Control 123, DOI 10.1007/978-3-319-65012-8_6

Fig. 6.1 The refining
concepts in EDO

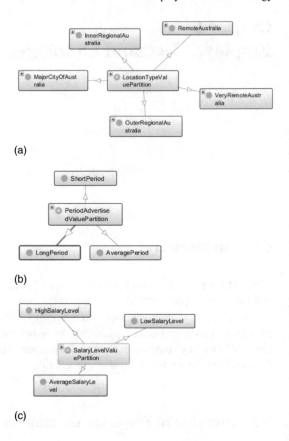

Western Australia, Australia's largest geographical state, where Perth is the capital
city.

The EDO has refining/dependent concepts which are value types and values
which partition conceptual spaces. Figure 6.1 illustrates the refining concepts. The
dependent concepts are the concepts of

- location type (inner regional Australia, major city of Australia, outer regional
  Australia, remote Australia, very remote Australia) as shown in Fig. 6.1a,
- period advertised (average, long, short) as shown in Fig. 6.1b, and
- salary level (average, high, low) as shown in Fig. 6.1c.

EDO has been developed in Web Ontology Language (OWL) using Protégé 5.0. It
contains 3615 logical axioms, 200 classes, 31 object properties, 7 data properties
and 1723 instances. The EDO has been reasoned to check its logical consistency.
The FaCT++, HermiT, Pellet, Pellet (Incremental), RacerPro and TrOWL reasoners
were all used for consistency verification. The reasoners checked the class, object
property and data property hierarchies, the class assertions, the object property
assertions and whether there were the same individuals contained within the

ontology. Consistency verification through a reasoner for EDO included consistency checking, concept satisfiability, classification, and realisation. These facilities are all standard inference services conventionally provided by a reasoner. EDO does not contain any contradictory facts—logical consistency of the ontology was also checked through the reasoners mentioned above. EDO also has the concept 'satisfiability', i.e. a class in the EDO is able to have instances. Defining an instance of a class causes the whole ontology to be inconsistent if a class is unsatisfiable. EDO also has a complete class hierarchy (classification service) that can be used to answer queries. The most specific class that an instance belongs to can be found in EDO (realisation service). From this verification experiment, EDO was found to be consistent and ready for user consumption.

6.3   EDO Classes

EDO classes are representations of employer demand concepts. They are described by formal descriptions stating precisely the conditions for membership of each class. Occupational types conceptualised in EDO are defined under the Australian and New Zealand Standard Classification of Occupations (ANZSCO). Figure 6.2 shows the EDO classes and its subclasses. As an example, the type of applicant requirements indicated as necessary for a vacancy in EDO are *Attribute Requirements*, *CompetenceRequirements* and *OtherRequirements*.

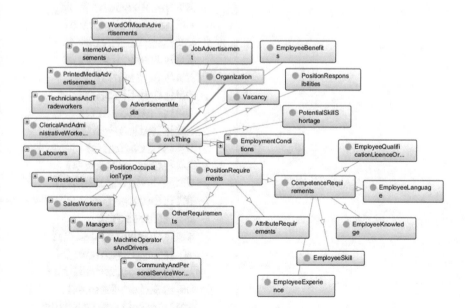

Fig. 6.2 EDO classes and its subclasses

6.4   Object and Data Properties

EDO object properties are relationship between employer demand classes or
employer demand instances; that is, properties can link either two employer demand
concepts or two employer demand occupational instances together. For example, the
property *hasEmployer* links the class *JobAdvertisement* with the class *Organization*
but also links the instance *MW1* (an instance of the class *Job Advertisement*) to the
instance *IPA Healthcare* (an instance of the class *Organization*). Figure 6.3 shows
the EDO object properties.

Fig. 6.3   EDO object
properties

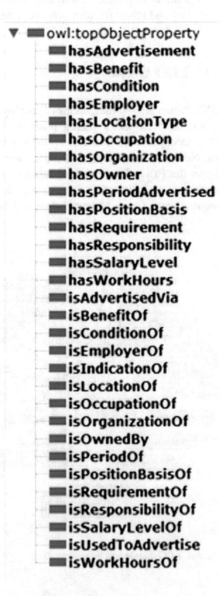

▼ ■ owl:topObjectProperty
　■ hasAdvertisement
　■ hasBenefit
　■ hasCondition
　■ hasEmployer
　■ hasLocationType
　■ hasOccupation
　■ hasOrganization
　■ hasOwner
　■ hasPeriodAdvertised
　■ hasPositionBasis
　■ hasRequirement
　■ hasResponsibility
　■ hasSalaryLevel
　■ hasWorkHours
　■ isAdvertisedVia
　■ isBenefitOf
　■ isConditionOf
　■ isEmployerOf
　■ isIndicationOf
　■ isLocationOf
　■ isOccupationOf
　■ isOrganizationOf
　■ isOwnedBy
　■ isPeriodOf
　■ isPositionBasisOf
　■ isRequirementOf
　■ isResponsibilityOf
　■ isSalaryLevelOf
　■ isUsedToAdvertise
　■ isWorkHoursOf

Fig. 6.4 EDO data properties

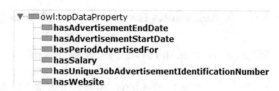

Figure 6.4 shows the EDO data properties. Below shows the data properties relates class or individual with data values.

- The data property *hasAdvertisementEndDate* relates a class or an individual with XML Schema Datatype of *date Time*.
- The data property *hasAdvertisementStartDate* relates a class or an individual with XML Schema Datatype of *date Time*.
- The data property *hasPeriodAdvertisedFor* relates a class or an individual with XML Schema Datatype of *integer*.
- The data property *hasSalary* relates a class or an individual with XML Schema Datatype of *integer*.
- The data property *hasUniqueJobAdvertisementIdentificationNumber* relates a class or an individual with XML Schema Datatype of *integer*.
- The data property *hasWebsite* relates a class or an individual with XML Schema Datatype of *any URI*.

6.5   Instance Populations

Employer demand instances can generally be referred to as individual members of specific classes that represent objects in the employer demand domain. These instances can have properties related to them that further define their existence. For example, in the employer demand domain, the class *JobAdvertisement* holds many instances that are specific occurrences of a job advertisement in the employer demand domain. Figure 6.5 shows 7 instances of class *JobAdvertisement* for Nurse Educators and Researchers advertisements.

Fig. 6.5 EDO instances of class *JobAdvertisement*

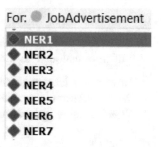

6.6   Applications for Employer Demand Ontology

EDO can be used to advance existing eRecruitment and eHumanResources applications. In this section, we demonstrate four fictional use cases based on stakeholders. These use cases have been formulated from real-world usage examples to show the applications for employer demand identification. For every use case, we present with scenario, questions, and queries and results. In order to query for the use cases, the Description Logic (DL) Query in Protégé has been used.

6.6.1   Government Official Developing Policy and Funding Protocols

Scenario

Thomas works at the Department of Health in Perth as the State Manager: Workforce Development. His area is responsible for looking after the whole of Western Australia's health staffing supply needs. This includes issues like ensuring that there are enough doctors in each town to serve the community; that colleges and vocational institutions have sufficient funding; to ensure students are trained in the occupational areas of need so there is sufficient supply of staff across the state; and to assign grants to groups that are able and keen to manage projects that can support the work that the Department of Health is doing towards their state-wide workforce management responsibilities. One of the tasks that Thomas looks after on a quarterly basis, is to draw up an environmental scan of the health workforce in Western Australia, to inform his area's policy development practices. Among other tasks, he telephones companies to enquire about recent skill shortages experienced over the last three months and looks at the job boards online to get a feel for the number of job advertisements and types of occupations that employers are advertising at that point in time. This informs his analysis and subsequent report writing. However, Thomas is finding it increasingly difficult to make an informed judgement about the vacancies—the job boards do not provide detailed analyses about the number and types of jobs for each regional area, nor does he have the time to trawl each advertisement to get more information, and keep track of the number of advertisements being posted online every day.

Questions

To assist Thomas in his quest, he would like to access EDO to obtain the following type of information from the system:

1. How many jobs were advertised in total for Regional and Remote Areas in Western Australia compared to those advertised for Perth's Metropolitan area?
2. Which nursing occupation group had the most requirements from employers?

Queries and Results

The above questions in natural language are formulated into DL query language as follows.

1. How many jobs were advertised in total for Regional and Remote Areas in Western Australia compared to those advertised for Perth's Metropolitan area?

For this question, two queries need to be run—one for each of the two areas specified. The first query which depicts in Fig. 6.6 is made to retrieve all the job advertisement instances that were advertised for Perth's Metropolitan area. The query result shows 80 instances.

The second query which depicts in Fig. 6.7 is made to retrieve all the job advertisement instances that were advertised for Western Australia's Regional and Remote areas. The query result shows 4 instances.

It is clear that many more positions were being advertised for Western Australia's metropolitan area than for any regional areas in Australia. This contradicts reports read in the literature, where it is always indicated that a greater number of vacancies exist in regional areas than in metropolitan areas, and this is an issue Thomas should be investigating.

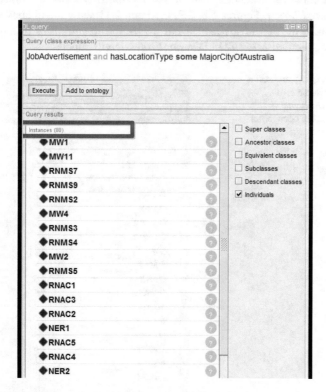

Fig. 6.6 DL Query and result showing the number of *JobAdvertisements* advertised in Western Australia's metropolitan area

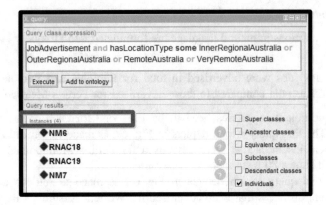

Fig. 6.7 DL Query and result showing the number of *JobAdvertisements* advertised in Western Australia's regional areas

2. Which nursing occupation group had the most requirements from employers?

For this question, four queries need to be run—one for each type of nursing occupation class i.e. *Midwives*, *NurseEducatorsAndResearchers*, *NurseManagers* and *RegisteredNurses*. Figures 6.8, 6.9, 6.10 and 6.11 show the queries to retrieve answers where the *JobAdvertisement* has a *Position Requirement* of any type for each of the specified *MidwifeAndNursingProfessionals* subclasses.

Fig. 6.8 DL Query and result showing the number of *PositionRequirements* advertised for the occupation class *Midwives*

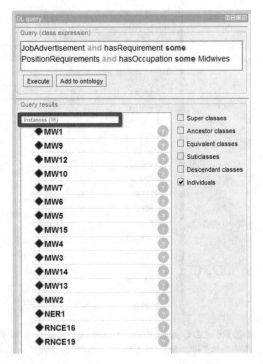

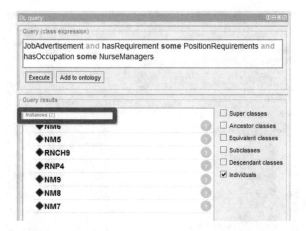

Fig. 6.9 DL Query and result showing the number of *PositionRequirements* advertised for the occupation class *NurseManagers*

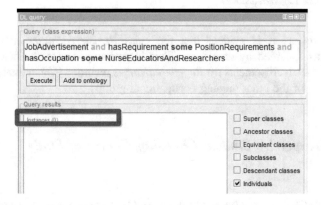

Fig. 6.10 DL Query and result showing the number of *PositionRequirements* advertised for the occupation class *NurseEducatorsAndResearchers*

The results for the four queries are as follows:

- The class *Midwives* had 16 instances where *Position Requirements* were advertised by employers.
- The class *Nurse Managers* had 7 instances where *Position Requirements* were advertised by employers.
- The class *Nurse Educators And Researchers* had 0 instances where *Position Requirements* were advertised by employers.
- The class *RegisteredNurses* had 64 instances where *PositionRequirements* were advertised by employers.

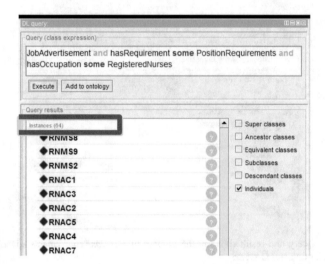

Fig. 6.11 DL Query and result showing the number of *PositionRequirements* advertised for the occupation class R*egisteredNurses*

From the results it is evident that the class *RegisteredNurses* had the most requirements specified by employers. This is probably due to the fact that there were far more advertisements for *RegisteredNurses* recorded (67) in total, than there were for any of the other nursing occupational groups.

6.6.2 Prospective Student Choosing Course of Study

Scenario

Sophi has finished her final year of school, and is about to submit her application to further her studies at one of the local universities in Perth. As her grandmother was an inspiration to Sophi all her life, Sophi has decided to follow in her footsteps and also become a Midwife who could look after those in need. Sophi has determined that two universities in Perth offer nursing as a course to study, however these universities do not provide the same areas of specialisation in nursing, and Sophi is unsure which nursing specialisation she needs to apply for (and hence which university), to pursue her goal. Sophi has had a fond relationship with her grandmother and all her grandmother's friends in the old age home where her grandmother spent her last years, but is more keen on caring for pregnant mothers and their babies than becoming a Registered Nurse in Aged Care. This has made Sophi wonder which attribute requirements employers are looking for when recruiting Midwifes, and also Nurse Managers, so she can apply for the nursing degree that best suits her personality and interests, but also will land her a job once she finishes with university.

Questions

To assist Sophi in her quest, she would like to access EDO to obtain the following type of information from the system:

1. What are the attribute requirements that employers are looking for when employing Midwifes?
2. What are the attribute requirements that employers are looking for when employing Nurse Managers?

Queries and Results

The above questions in natural language are formulated into DL query language as follows.

1. What are the attribute requirements that employers are looking for when employing Midwifes?

The question requires two steps to be performed. Firstly the DL Query which depicts in Fig. 6.12 is made to retrieve all *JobAdvertisement* instances advertised for Midwives where any type of *AttributeRequirements* was specified. The query result returns 3 job advertisements. The second step requires to look at each of job advertisements provided in the query result and the specific attribute requirements can be investigated. Job advertisement *MW6*, shows that the attribute requirements *Caring* and *ConfidentialityCommitment* were listed in the job advertisement as requirements that prospective applicants of that vacancy should have. *MW3* required prospective applicants to have Enthusiasm, and *MW3* required prospective applicants to have *CustomerServiceCommitment*.

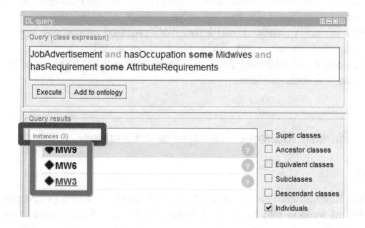

Fig. 6.12 DL Query and result showing the *JobAdvertisement* instances that were advertised for the occupation class *Midwives* where a type of *AttributeRequirement* was specified

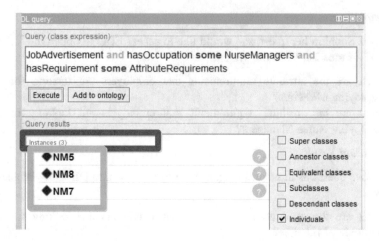

Fig. 6.13 DL Query and result showing the *JobAdvertisement* instances that were advertised for the occupation class *NurseManagers* where a type of *AttributeRequirement* was specified

2. What are the attribute requirements that employers are looking for when employing Nurse Managers?

This question requires two steps to be performed. Firstly the DL Query which depicts in Fig. 6.13 is made to retrieve all *JobAdvertisement* instances advertised for *NurseManagers* where any type of *AttributeRequirements* were specified. The query result return 3 job advertisements. The second step requires to look at each of job advertisements provided in the query result and the specific attribute requirements can be investigated. Job advertisement *NM5* shows that the attribute requirements *DeliveringExcellence*, *FlexibleToChangingResidentNeeds* and Enthusiasm, were listed in the job advertisement as requirements prospective applicants of that vacancy should have. *NM7* required prospective applicants to have *RelateToDementia*, and *NM8* required prospective applicants to have *Proactive* and *CanDoAttitude*. From the above information, Sophi is able to do a comparison and make decision.

6.6.3   Human Resource Manager at a Company

Scenario

Anita is a Recruitment Advisor at the New Perth Hospital, which is currently being expanded to include two brand new areas for the hospital: maternity ward and community health day visit facilities. The two new wings of the building will be completed and ready for operation in approximately six months' time, at which stage staff will be employed to cover for these new areas of operation. Anita is trying to establish what the market is offering to midwives and community health nurses in terms of employee benefits. This is so that she can ensure the New Perth Hospital will be competitive in the staff packages that they would like to advertise in their job advertisements, thus guaranteeing they get a sufficient number of applications for the many positions she needs to fill. At this point in time, Anita does not have the time to analyse each job advertisement one-by-one for the last month, to obtain this type of information from the job advertisements' free text sections.

Questions

To assist Anita in her quest, she would like to access EDO to obtain the following type of information from the system:

1. What type of employee benefits have been offered to Midwives and Nurse Professionals in the Perth metropolitan area?
2. How many employers are prepared to offer Visa Sponsorships to their prospective candidates?

Queries and Results

The above questions in natural language are formulated into DL query language as follows.

1. What type of employee benefits have been offered to Midwives and Nurse Professionals in the Perth metropolitan area?

For this question, DL query need to run as shown in Fig. 6.14 to retrieve all job advertisements where the location has been included as a *MajorCityOfAustralia*. The query result shows 54 instances or job advertisements which included

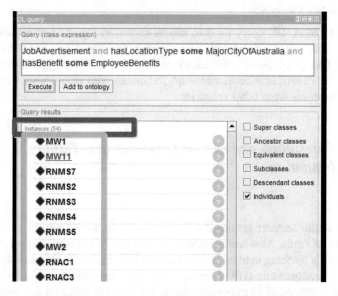

Fig. 6.14 DL Query and result showing the JobAdvertisement instances that were advertised for all nursing occupation classes where a type of AttributeRequirement was specified

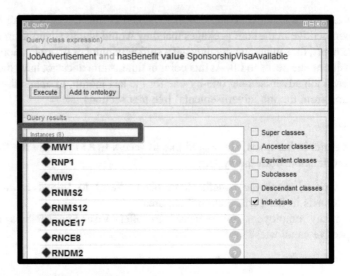

Fig. 6.15 DL Query and result showing the *JobAdvertisement* instances that specified the employee benefit *SponsorshipVisaAvailable*

employee benefits. It is clear to Anita that many employers offer *SponsorshipVisaAvailable*, *ProfessionalDevelopment*, *SalaryPackaging*, etc. and as such will consider offering these benefits to their future employees, as the minimum to be able to attract top calibre applicants.

2. How many employers are prepared to offer Visa Sponsorships to their prospective candidates?

For this question, DL query need to run as shown in Fig. 6.15 to retrieve all job advertisements where sponsorship visas have been offered as part of the position package. The query result indicates to Anita that a total of 8 job advertisements included the benefit of visa sponsorships for nurses who would want to come and work in Australia from other countries.

6.6.4 Curriculum and Career Developer at a Tertiary Institution

Scenario

Carl is a senior lecturer in Surgical Practices 410 in the Faculty of Health at the University of Perth. As a senior lecturer, one of Carl's responsibilities is to ensure that his unit's teaching content is relevant to what employers are currently looking for, in terms of graduate skill capabilities. He also needs to ensure that students are accurately informed of all the qualifications that they are expected to have once they have completed their nursing degrees at the University of Perth. Before students are

able to graduate from the University of Perth's Nursing degree, they are sent for
in-house practical training as part of the university's agreement with the New Perth
Hospital. During their practical training period, students are able to attend additional courses at the New Perth Hospital. This is part of the university's commitment to help students land a job at their employer of choice as soon as they have
completed their practical work. The students are keen to know which employers of
the top three hospitals in Perth were the largest advertiser of vacancies, so that they
can direct their job seeking efforts towards those institutions.

Questions

To assist Carl in his quest, he would like to access EDO to obtain the following type
of information from the system:

1. What types of skill requirements are employers indicating they need when
   employing Registered Nurses?
2. Which of the top three hospitals in Perth was the major employer during January
   2011?

Queries and Results

The above questions in natural language are formulated into DL query language as
follows.

1. What types of skill requirements are employers indicating they need when
   employing Registered Nurses?

For this question, DL query need to run as shown in Fig. 6.16 to retrieve all job
advertisement instances in which employee skills were listed as a requirement for
applicants. The query result returns 29 job advertisements which include some type

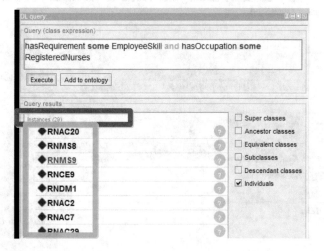

Fig. 6.16 DL Query and result showing some of the *JobAdvertisement* instances that specified
employee skills as a requirement

of employee skills as a requirement. It is then necessary to follow the identified job advertisements to see which employee skill requirements were listed in each of the relevant job advertisements. It is clear to Carl that employers seem to regularly require applicants to have *GoodCommunicationSkills*, *TeamPlayerSkills*, *WorkUnsupervisedSkills*, etc.

2. Which of the top three hospitals in Perth was the major employer?

This question requires three DL Queries to be run—one for each top hospital in Perth as shown in Figs. 6.17, 6.18 and 6.19.

   From the query results it would seem that both *MercyHospital* and *StJohnOfGodSubiaco* advertised three positions while *BethesdaHospital* only advertised for two positions.

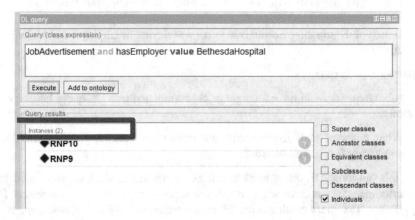

Fig. 6.17 DL Query and result showing the number of job advertisements the employer *BethesdaHospital* advertised

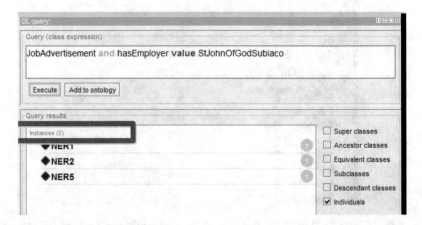

Fig. 6.18 DL Query and result showing the number of job advertisements the employer *StJohnOfGodSubiaco* advertised

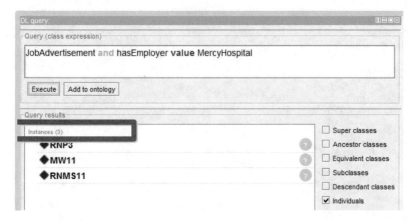

Fig. 6.19 DL Query and result showing the number of job advertisements the employer *MercyHospital* advertised

6.7   Conclusion

This chapter is an integral part of employer demand identification as presented in the EDO, the backbone to the framework. The chapter has provided EDO structure and its usage in case studies. Integration and augmentation of PPAC and EDO for healthcare and workforce management systems can be achieved via the following:

- A new class named *CulturallyCompetentHealthcarePositionRequirement* which has sub classes

  - *CapabilityCulturallyandLinguisticallyDisadvantagedPatients* which has properties e.g. hasSpecificCulturalType (i.e. culturally and linguistically diverse (CALD) ethnicities)
  - *ChronicDiseaseCareTrained*
  - *ChronicDiseaseExperienced*
  - *ChronicDiseaseHealthcareType*
  - *TrainableforChronicDiseaseHealthcareType*.

Difference illustrated here is that when recruiting it will be necessary to accept that not all applicants are experienced and may be put off when the recruiting entity is desperate.

Reference

Smalberger, C.: An Employer Demand Intelligence Framework. http://espace.library.curtin.edu.au/
   R?func=dbin-jump-full&local_base=gen01-era02&object_id=199399 (2013)

Chapter 7
Employer Demand Intelligence

7.1 Introduction

It is very important to have a clear picture of the job market at any time—not only for governments for timely decision making but also for scenarios like individuals doing career planning. Furthermore, due to the volatile and dynamic nature of the job market it is essential that the information about employer demand is up-to-date. This information can be collected from job advertisements and published on the web. However, the job advertisements usually contain unstructured information in textual form, with frequent usage of specific jargon related to the nature and field of the advertised vacancy. Additionally, the information collection involves hundreds of advertisements, which is difficult to process manually, if possible at all. The advertisements, albeit highly unstructured, are already in digital form and the development of an automated process capable of extracting meaningful structured data and statistics for these text advertisements can be extremely useful in this scenario. In this chapter we present development of a semi-automated Employer Demand Intelligence Tool (EDIT). The fine detailed development of EDIT can be found in Terblanche and Wongthongtham (2015).

7.2 Introduction of Employer Demand Intelligence Tool

EDIT has been developed around the EDO in order to semi-automatically populate and enhance EDO based on the content of online-published job advertisements. EDIT functionality is as follows:

- Extract job advertisement content from html text by filtering unwanted web content.
- Recognise the existence of concepts found in the online job advertisements that match with those concepts stored in EDO.

© Springer International Publishing AG 2018
D.E. Forbes et al., *Ontology Engineering Applications in Healthcare and Workforce Management Systems*, Studies in Systems, Decision and Control 123, DOI 10.1007/978-3-319-65012-8_7

- Provide the ability to link the recognised text to the corresponding concept in EDO.
- Develop the ability to populate job advertisement instances for EDO and assert relevant object and datatype property values.

Input of EDIT is those job advertisements collected in their original HTML format for Western Australian locations, and for the Nursing and Midwifery occupations only and output is the Populated and evolved/enhanced EDO and dataset. EDIT has been designed to gather data from unstructured text on the web (social media, company, government and other websites) by utilising ontology-assisted information extraction techniques.

7.3   System Architecture

The main processes of EDIT for its development is presented in Fig. 7.1.

The process starts where EDIT collects and stores the information from the job board SEEK for occupations under the Registered Nurse and Midwifery classification into EDIT's corpus. Unnecessary web page content such as links to other pages and graphics is removed and only the advertisement content is stored in the corpus. The next process entails the extraction of information contained in the corpus, where the useful information which matches with the concepts in EDO, is extracted from the advertisement text. In addition to the corpus creation process, the process also uses a gazetteer, which is the output (called the EDO domain knowledge) of another process. This process extracts the concepts (classes and instances) in EDO and stores them in the gazetteer. The gazetteer is a standard term in the area of text processing to store entity names or nouns. Finally, the

Fig. 7.1 Main processes of the EDIT

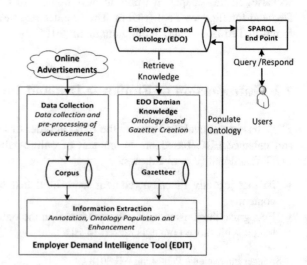

information extracted from each advertisement is populated into the ontology or used to add extra components to EDO—no concepts are deleted or removed from EDO. The data relating to the generic concepts of EDO are populated into EDO as instances and property values. This extended ontology forms the knowledge base which end users can query via the SPARQL endpoint, in order to obtain answers for their employer demand intelligence interrogations.

7.4 Case Study

When the framework recognises the occurrence of concepts in the job advertisements, matching those contained in EDO, it creates an instance for each advertisement in the EDO. After this, the additional concepts recognised are linked to the instance of the advertisement, using object properties and datatype properties. The system has the ability to create new datatype or object properties in the ontology for those instances for which there is no matching or appropriate property. As such, an enhanced ontology evolves alongside the ontology population process.

A case study is provided to illustrate the processes that a single job advertisement undergoes during the different stages of the framework.

7.4.1 Data Collection

An example of a typical job advertisement archived from seek.com as collected in the first step is provided in Fig. 7.2. In addition to advertisement related content, web pages also have links to other pages on the website which are removed in the pre-processing stage to get a simplified advertisement as shown in Fig. 7.3.

7.4.2 Loading the Advertisement as a Corpus

All the advertisements are loaded as a corpus language resource into the GATE system as shown in Fig. 7.4.

7.4.3 EDIT Pipeline

In this step the EDIT pipeline performs the following seven processes on the advertisement.

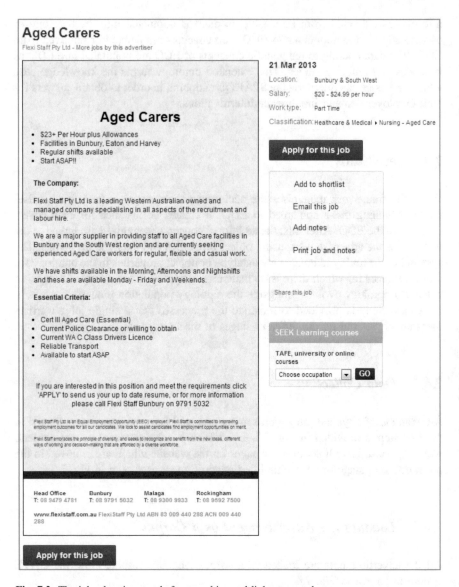

Fig. 7.2 The job advertisement before graphics and links removed

1. Document Reset: This process clears the results of any previous execution of the pipeline on a document and refreshes the system for the next processes.
2. Tokenization: This process breaks up the text into tokens as shown in Fig. 7.5a.
3. Sentence splitting: In this stage, the sentence boundaries are determined as shown in Fig. 7.5b.

---

21 Mar 2013

- Location:
  Bunbury & South West

- Salary:
  $20 - $24.99 per hour

- Work type:
  Part Time

- Classification:
  Healthcare & Medical Nursing - Aged Care

Aged Carers

- $23+ Per Hour plus Allowances
- Facilities in Bunbury, Eaton and Harvey
- Regular shifts available
- Start ASAP!!

The Company:

Flexi Staff Pty Ltd is a leading Western Australian owned and managed company specialising in all aspects of the recruitment and labour hire.

We are a major supplier in providing staff to all Aged Care facilities in Bunbury and the South West region and are currently seeking experienced Aged Care workers for regular, flexible and casual work.

We have shifts available in the Morning, Afternoons and Nightshifts and these are available Monday - Friday and Weekends.

Essential Criteria:

- Cert III Aged Care (Essential)
- Current Police Clearance or willing to obtain
- Current WA C Class Drivers Licence
- Reliable Transport
- Available to start ASAP

Fig. 7.3 The job advertisement after graphics and links removed

4. POS tagging and morphological Analysis: The results of these two steps are show in Fig. 7.6. POS tagging determines the usage of a word (noun, verb etc.) and the morphological analyser find the root word (e.g. manage for managed).
5. Recognition of concepts appearing in the text by the flexible gazetteer as shown in Fig. 7.7.
6. The word-list based gazetteer along with the "JAPE Transducer Text" is used to recognise salary amounts and dates appearing in the text as information about these is not available in EDO.
7. The information extracted by the previous steps is populated into EDO by creating a knowledge instance for the advertisement with properties shown in Fig. 7.8.

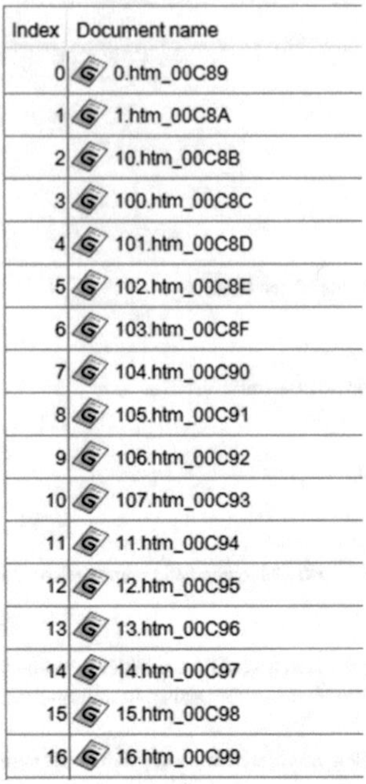

Index	Document name
0	0.htm_00C89
1	1.htm_00C8A
2	10.htm_00C8B
3	100.htm_00C8C
4	101.htm_00C8D
5	102.htm_00C8E
6	103.htm_00C8F
7	104.htm_00C90
8	105.htm_00C91
9	106.htm_00C92
10	107.htm_00C93
11	11.htm_00C94
12	12.htm_00C95
13	13.htm_00C96
14	14.htm_00C97
15	15.htm_00C98
16	16.htm_00C99

Fig. 7.4 A collection of job advertisements loaded into corpus

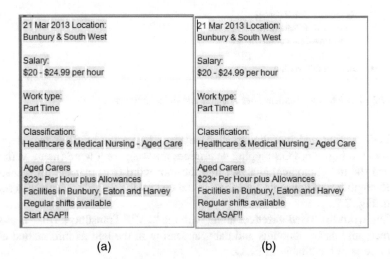

(a)   (b)

Fig. 7.5 The job advertisement is breaking into tokens and then being sentence split

category=DT, kind=word, length=1, orth=lowercase, root=a, string=a}

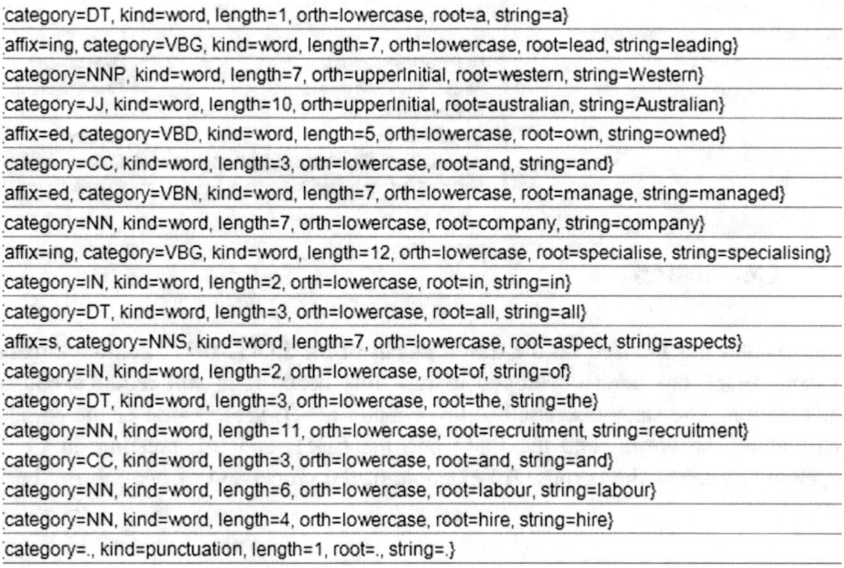

affix=ing, category=VBG, kind=word, length=7, orth=lowercase, root=lead, string=leading}

category=NNP, kind=word, length=7, orth=upperInitial, root=western, string=Western}

category=JJ, kind=word, length=10, orth=upperInitial, root=australian, string=Australian}

affix=ed, category=VBD, kind=word, length=5, orth=lowercase, root=own, string=owned}

category=CC, kind=word, length=3, orth=lowercase, root=and, string=and}

affix=ed, category=VBN, kind=word, length=7, orth=lowercase, root=manage, string=managed}

category=NN, kind=word, length=7, orth=lowercase, root=company, string=company}

affix=ing, category=VBG, kind=word, length=12, orth=lowercase, root=specialise, string=specialising}

category=IN, kind=word, length=2, orth=lowercase, root=in, string=in}

category=DT, kind=word, length=3, orth=lowercase, root=all, string=all}

affix=s, category=NNS, kind=word, length=7, orth=lowercase, root=aspect, string=aspects}

category=IN, kind=word, length=2, orth=lowercase, root=of, string=of}

category=DT, kind=word, length=3, orth=lowercase, root=the, string=the}

category=NN, kind=word, length=11, orth=lowercase, root=recruitment, string=recruitment}

category=CC, kind=word, length=3, orth=lowercase, root=and, string=and}

category=NN, kind=word, length=6, orth=lowercase, root=labour, string=labour}

category=NN, kind=word, length=4, orth=lowercase, root=hire, string=hire}

category=., kind=punctuation, length=1, root=., string=.}

Fig. 7.6 POS and morphological checking of the job advertisement

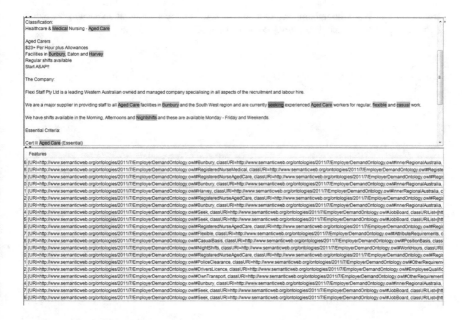

Fig. 7.7 The EDO based gazetteer recognises the concepts in the advertisement text

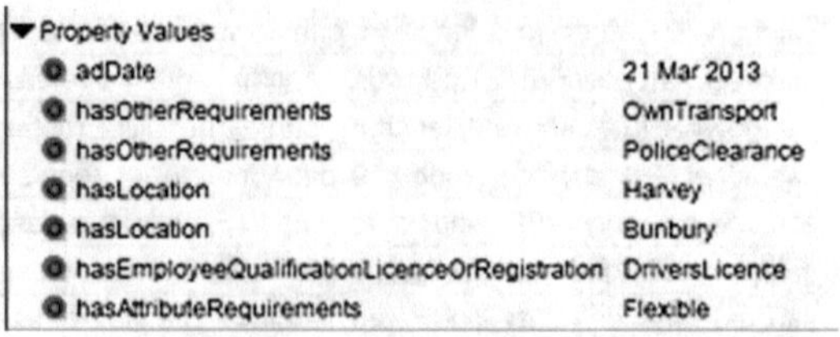

Fig. 7.8 Extracted
information is populated into
EDO

▼ Property Values	
● adDate	21 Mar 2013
● hasOtherRequirements	OwnTransport
● hasOtherRequirements	PoliceClearance
● hasLocation	Harvey
● hasLocation	Bunbury
● hasEmployeeQualificationLicenceOrRegistration	DriversLicence
● hasAttributeRequirements	Flexible

7.5   Conclusion

This chapter has focused on the development of the EDIT. It is a semi-automatic
system; EDIT has been developed at run time hence it is still requires human
intervention. The steps discussed in this chapter are (i) the creation of the corpus,
(ii) loading the corpus and the EDO into the EDIT, and (iii) creating an EDIT
pipeline to process the corpus. An example of the processing of one job has been
provided.

Reference

Terblanche, C., Wongthongtham, P.: Ontology-based employer demand management. Softw.
    Pract. Exp. http://onlinelibrary.wiley.com/doi/10.1002/spe.2319/pdf (2015)

Chapter 8
Intelligent System

8.1 Introduction

Ontologies play an important role in enabling knowledge representation, knowledge management, and knowledge sharing. Many applications benefit greatly from making use of ontologies as a means of achieving semantic interoperability among heterogeneous and distributed systems. They are considered as one of the key enablers for the emerging Semantic Web by making the Web content accessible to humans and computers (Li et al. 2005). Ontologies are in a machine understandable and processable format, thereby enabling the software agents to understand the contents autonomously. Therefore, the integration of ontologies and multi-agent systems, also known as the ontology-based multi-agent approach, allows software applications to benefit from both technologies. For instance, ontologies can assist with data retrieval, while the agents can act as autonomous software entities that can interact with the environment and with other agents (Garanina et al. 2013). In this chapter, the integration of ontologies and multi-agent systems is focused.

8.2 Ontology-based Multi-agent Systems

It is evident that considerable efforts have been put into the integration of ontologies and multi-agent systems, also known as 'ontology-based multi-agent' approaches in order to dissimilate the knowledge captured in ontologies. Furthermore, some researchers have mentioned them as a means of facilitating knowledge assimilation by capturing and incorporating the knowledge into the ontology knowledge base. These works encompass various domains including software engineering, health, education, e-commerce, finance, etc. Table 8.1 provides a summary of the aforementioned ontology-based multi-agent systems.

© Springer International Publishing AG 2018   87
D.E. Forbes et al., *Ontology Engineering Applications in Healthcare and Workforce Management Systems*, Studies in Systems, Decision and Control 123, DOI 10.1007/978-3-319-65012-8_8

Table 8.1 Review of some existing ontology-based multi-agent systems

Application Domain	Source	Objectives of ontology-based multi-agent systems	Purpose of agent's use of ontology
Software Engineering	Monte-Alto et al. (2012)	Process contextual information and support human resource allocation	– Contextual information retrieval – Knowledge reasoning
	Teixeira and Huzita (2014)	Support human resource allocation in globally distributed software projects	– Information retrieval – Knowledge reasoning – Knowledge manipulation
Health	Wang et al. (2010)	Evaluate the health of diets	– Represent personal profile and food model – Information analysis
	Li and Mackaness (2015)	Enhance the performance of Epidemiology information retrieval in a dynamic decision-making environment	– Information retrieval – Spatial and temporal reasoning
Education	Oriche et al. (2013)	Automate the semantic annotation of educational resources	– Assign domain knowledge to educational resources
E-commerce	Yang et al. (2007)	Support communication, interaction, and management among different parties engaged in the accommodation e-market	– Facilitate agent communication – Describe agent services
Finance	Ying et al. (2013)	Automate some market analysis tasks	– Represent financial domain knowledge – Facilitate agent's communication and collaboration

Monte-Alto et al. (2012) and Teixeira and Huzita (2014) propose a context processing mechanism called ContextP-GSD (Context Processing on Global Software Development) that utilises contextual information to assist users during the software development process. This mechanism applies agent-based technology to process contextual information and support human resource allocation.

Wang et al. (2010) introduce an ontology-based multi-agent system for intelligent healthcare applications to assist users to evaluate diets. The ontologies have been developed to represent personal profiles and food models. Agents use these ontologies to analyse appropriate diet information based on a user profile.

Li and Mackaness (2015) develop a system that is based on a multi-agent architecture to support decision-making for epidemic management. The system is intended to enhance the performance of information retrieval in a dynamic decision making environment. Inexperienced personnel can use this system to locate online data and to process services for spatio-temporal analysis of a specified environmental epidemic. Ontologies for dataset and service semantics are used to describe general concepts of GIS web service and epidemiology data management, while lightweight ontologies for simple spatial and temporal reasoning are used to add spatial and temporal semantics to the geospatial data. The agents utilise these ontologies to enable automated semantic service discovery and composition.

Oriche et al. (2013) propose a semantic annotation system based on three main agents to manage the semantic annotation of educational resources. These agents utilise the domain ontology to assign domain knowledge to learning objects. Once these resources have been annotated, they are conceptualised and organised well so that they can be delivered to the users on demand according to their profiles and needs.

Yang et al. (2007) introduce an ontology-based multi-agent system for the accommodation services industry to support the online accommodation market. The domain ontology is used to facilitate agent communication and collaboration as well as the development of an ontology-based data transformation mechanism for data structure translation.

Ying et al. (2013) introduce MOMA, a framework for creating ontology-based multi-agent systems, and incorporated an experiment in financial application development. MOMA consists of two main development phases: ontology development and agent development. However, the researchers focus only on the development of ontology and the use of the ontology to drive the implementation of the agent application. The agent development part is treated as a black box, but no details are provided regarding the design of the agent's application. The agents make use of the ontology to facilitate consistent inter-agent communication and coordination.

8.3   The Integration of Ontologies and Software Agents

The benefits of both technologies can be had by integrating ontology and software agents. Ontology is used for knowledge representation, knowledge integration, knowledge sharing and reuse. The features of the software agent and multi-agent system, such as autonomy, reactivity, pro-activeness, social ability, adaptability and dynamism, provide a potential solution for applications that are complex, dynamic and distributed. Therefore, they can be deployed in the application if only one of the approaches cannot satisfactorily resolve the problem. As the ontology and agent-based technology address different aspects of the same problem, they complement each other.

In recent years, the ontology-based multi-agent approach has attracted considerable interest in research. As presented and discussed in the previous section regarding the state-of-the-art ontology-based multi-agent systems, the majority of research has focused on the use of ontology to facilitate agents' communication, represent domain knowledge and help to locate and retrieve information, and reasoning the knowledge.

8.3.1   Facilitating Agents' Communication

In a multi-agent system, each agent usually cooperates with other agents to achieve a common goal; therefore, it needs the ability to communicate and interact with other agents by exchanging messages. The agent communication languages such as KQML and FIPA-ACL specify the syntax of the exchange messages but not the semantics of the messages. In this case, ontology can be additionally supplied in the messages to formalise the semantics of the exchanged message in a format that is understandable by agents in order to facilitate consistent communication and interoperability.

8.3.2   Representing Domain Knowledge and Helping to Locate and Retrieve Information

Ontology can be used to describe domain knowledge and information content which is pertinent to that domain. With the use of ontologies in MAS, domain knowledge does not need to be embedded within the agents. Therefore, it creates an opportunity to share and reuse the domain knowledge and also has the potential to reuse the MAS infrastructure for other applications. Moreover, software agents have the ability to read and understand knowledge captured in ontologies. Therefore, they are able to locate and retrieve the information requested by their user.

8.3.3   Reasoning the Knowledge

The use of ontologies coupled with MAS can support knowledge representation and reasoning capabilities of software applications that are developed by deploying the MAS approach. The integration of ontologies in MAS can lead to the creation of logic rules that can be applied by a semantic reasoner to infer new knowledge not explicitly defined in ontologies (Freitas et al. 2015).

8.4   Employment Demands and Healthcare Service Delivery Management Systems

How can we estimate and plan for future employee staffing needs, as the 'future' constantly appears to reshape itself? Demand intelligence implicitly represents guesswork about the ever-unfolding needs of employers. The future is an intangible, unqualifiable and unquantifiable entity.

Disruptive, sudden, unexpected and powerful change, arriving predominantly in the form of techno-commercial innovation, is shortening the shelf-life of demand intelligence. Besides technological innovation, major shifts are forced upon us through unpredictable extremes such as wars and pandemics.

8.4.1   Uncertainty Affecting Physicians' Perspectives and Confidence

Simpkin and Schwartzstein (2016) refer to the discomfort of physicians through a "deep-rooted unwillingness' to tolerate uncertainty in their medical diagnostic deliberations, and that doctors continually have to make decisions on the basis of imperfect data and limited knowledge, which leads to uncertainty, coupled with the uncertainty that arises from unpredictable patient responses to treatment and from health care outcomes that are far from binary".

Rosendal et al. (2017) researching medically unexplained symptom disorders in primary care seek to establish greater certainty by concentrating on and proposing a new prognosis based-classification to view "the patient's risk of ongoing symptoms, complications, increased healthcare use or disability because of the symptoms".

Peter Curson is Emeritus Professor of Population and Health in the Faculty of Medicine and Health Sciences at Macquarie University and Honorary Professor of Population and Security at the University of Sydney. He is a prolific writer on research into population behavioural traits when nations are confronted by disasters like epidemics, pandemics and wars. His article in The Spectator Australia (Infections Persist, Pandemics Rule 2017) closed with two short sentences: "Many believe that future generations will have to face a dangerous array of infectious disease threats. It is a sobering thought".

8.4.2   A Study of the Implications for Culturally Competent Critical Healthcare Staffing

As a case study we imagine a vector-borne infectious disease epidemic occurring in the north of Australia, with many infected patients living among remote Aboriginal communities where English is not the first or even second, language. The rate of infection spread is alarmingly rapid and fairly soon people of varied ethnic family origin including culturally and linguistically disadvantaged migrant refugees begin to appear at suburban clinics and city hospital emergency departments. Many have no experience of Australian healthcare and the system is soon in danger of being overwhelmed. A contingency plan is brought into play once an alert has been announced nationally and an urgent search is undertaken to recruit and deploy health care workers with knowledge of and preferably experience in infectious disease care and diagnostic challenges such as those arising from medically unexplained symptoms (MUS). There is a danger of public panic as patients who have prior histories suffering from Myalgia Encephalomyelitis (ME)/Chronic Fatigue Syndrome (CFS) and Patients with longer term Lyme-like disease begin to suffer further debilitation.

In an imperfect resourcing scenario emergencies require some degree of compromise. Using an ontology driven assessment system, the EDI and PPAC combination will (a) enhance employee search quality and speed; and (b) radically improve prospects for finding health care practitioners with cultural competency strengths and thereby use these candidates as team leaders during the crisis; accepting that in the short term such skills will be in short supply. The PPAC concept, moving on from while adding to the type 2 diabetes domain, will enable field training to improve the quality of communication, and in time will become disease diagnosis and treatment specific. Once the information systems chain from physicians and pathology laboratories feeds into the frontline, identifying/classifying the sampled blood bacteria pathogen(s), those culturally competent and technically savvy leaders will be able to orchestrate real-time skills training updates within and across health care delivery teams.

The foregoing however does not dwell upon one serious barrier that persists in Australian healthcare, which is an ethos issue; the dogmatic resistance and controversial debate encircling tick-borne disease, notable under the Lyme-like description. The ensuing stigma, directed toward many patients and some caring General Practitioners, is largely perpetrated by influential sections of the health care fraternity. The stigma also surfaces just as vehemently in cases of MUS and ME/CFS. If such an epidemic with pandemic potential should occur now, in 2017, the government of Australia and the dominant professional healthcare leadership would most likely not possess the open, data-supported and trusted communications and information systems capabilities demanded by this scenario.

Smalberger (2013) devotes useful analysis to the subject of recruitment of nurses under the formal nomenclature headed by the title Registered Nurse, leading to a taxonomy of differing class subtitles. The pace of societal change and need for well-resourced response to epidemiological impacts, brings with it a constant call for new skills. Tomorrow's nursing and other healthcare recruit, qualified in the EDI ontology to aid the search through three requirements particularly—skills, attributes and location—will have to be found and employed through a different intelligence culture and data capture from today's methodology. The additional layers of skills and attributes, and the movement toward greater service mobility factoring will bring greater variety of properties into the ontology construct. For example, know-how in emerging diagnostics and treatments, ability to manage Australia's remote consultation and robotic treatment/surgery capabilities, and the advent of the 'researcher nurse' as a contributor to medical knowledge revisions, all represent potential job qualification ideals in the wording of advertisements and the automatic online application screening systems so commonly employed today.

From an ongoing review of recruitment practices and the inter-sector relationships between placement agencies, educational institutions, in-house training and accreditation systems in healthcare, we perceive that most especially in the context of emerging health care practices and the demand for cultural competence in a significantly multi-ethnic nation, the demand intelligence contribution by employers in the future will require greater initial flexibility. It will be less pedantic, more accommodating in recognition of the need to share the know-how pathway through workplace update and new skills training.

In the latter phase of research for this book many conversations with qualified and informed individuals have helped with our attempt to determine the most promising way to engage the broad array of stakeholders. Ultimately this is to be achieved by using human, natural language generated, and through computer aided intelligent reasoning, to understand and communicate successfully in medical consultations (PPIEs). Simultaneously we have digested many contributory sources in the peer-reviewed and open access literature; choosing not to include here the mass of references which are easily located via web searches.

Two primary considerations stand out. The first primary consideration is that Australian Aboriginal health has not made the progress desired as stated in the program Close the Gap introduced in 2008.

Questions are as follows:

What is the Australian experience in recruitment of culturally competent healthcare practitioners?

Are there any new trends emerging to show improved cultural competence (or the opposite) in our healthcare environment?

Is cultural diversity in Australia too complex for this to be treated as a holistic issue? (Especially considering the persistent presence of adverse outcomes in Aboriginal health).

Is it perhaps safer to assume that organisations that exist to train aspiring healthcare workers in cultural competence are Australia's best prospects, versus the time and cost of searching a very limited qualified market and/or sector employers accepting that time and cost of internal training after appointment?

Professor Sandra Thompson, Director, Western Australia Centre for Rural Health has a long history as a clinician whose research team is closely involved with Aboriginal Health. Thompson (2017) noted that over time and with the increased consciousness of Aboriginal disadvantage, there has been a lot more attention in the area, including the employment of Aboriginal people who are assumed to be able to do it well. There is also a lot more focus on training in the education pathway—although not always with evaluation of how well it works in changing attitudes and practices within the mainstream cultures within which people practise and also lots of online training these days. However how much people learn, retain and are influenced in their professional practice by it is largely unknown. At this point, at least in Western Australia, it is very aboriginal focussed possibly because the migrants are often Caucasian even if from other countries (e.g. New Zealand, South Africa, UK).

Thompson (2017) commented that one always has to take the longer term view and things are modestly improving, although up close it is so slow one feels not much is happening. The issue of investing in and training staff and the potential for them to go elsewhere is the continual issue that speaks to opportunities for promotion and a good workplace culture. In theory this should be ongoing trial and error.

Another comment from Richard Trudgen is reported here. Richard Trudgen has lived in North Arnhem Land for more than forty years, supporting the Yolŋu people through shared education and health knowledge development. His highly regarded book, cited in Forbes (2013) is close to unsurpassable in the explication of the conflict and inadequacies of the western medical culture in a minority ethnic (Aboriginal community) setting (Trudgen 2000). Forbes (2013) cited Trudgen (2000) as a very strong source of the data demonstrating pervasive cognitive dissonance in PPIEs involving Aboriginal patients and western-trained English speaking doctors. Discussing the continued poor state of health of the Yolŋu people, Richard commented in the context of medical consultations, of his encounters with European migrants who have told him that they too suffer hardship in health care due to the disjunctive experience in trying to engage with the Australian health care system.

For further exposition on this, (Gwynne and Lincoln 2016) identified evidence-based strategies in the literature for developing and maintaining a skilled and qualified rural and remote health workforce in Australia to meet the health care needs of Australian Aboriginal people.

The second primary consideration is that the diversity of cultures with the Australian nation is not and may never be, adequately accommodated in medical care terms given the population, demographics and logistics constraints of servicing people in and across a very large land mass with significant remote access characteristics. This drives the dual imperative; for developing ACTs such as the PPAC concept, and continually developing sophisticated succinctly-populated ontologies to ensure that the EDI system recognizes and responds to real-world achievable objectives.

8.4.3   Cognitive Computing and the Ontology Contributions

The IBM Watson 'supercomputer' Discovery Advisor work, in a review article by Chen et al. (2016) covers cognitive solutions, describing these as "trained to understand technical, industry-specific content and use advanced reasoning,

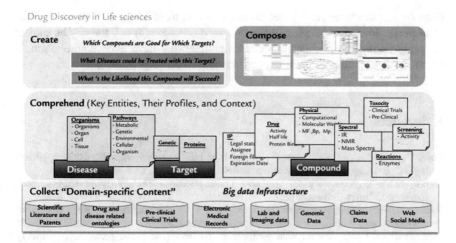

Fig. 8.1 Watson Discovery Advisor applied to life sciences (Chen et al. 2016)

predictive modelling, and machine and machine learning techniques to advance research faster". The article includes a very useful graphic illustration as shown in Fig. 8.1 showing Watson Discovery Advisor applied to Life Sciences.

In the 'Collect "Domain-specific Content"' it presents 'Drug and disease related ontologies'. In the body of text it states "Today, Watson Discovery Advisor for Life Sciences is supplied with dictionaries, thesauri, and ontologies on genes, proteins, drugs, and diseases. It includes annotators that are tested for accuracy in recognizing, extracting, and categorizing these entities". From this guidance we are reminded that substantial work is required to extensively draw upon and create greater granular value in building expanding and merging concept hierarchies in servicing and staffing of and for future healthcare.

8.5 Conclusion

Simplifying the case for resolving these two primary factors through synergic integration, we now look ahead to address the work that is required to elevate the goal of seeking finding and employing/deploying sufficiently versatile qualified and culturally competent health care workers, most particularly but not exclusively, nurses.

Ontology fed search agents will require expansive qualitative enrichment of hierarchical class, properties instances and relationships; the integration of validated ontology domains, and constantly improved empowerment of reasoning capabilities. Recruitment processes may need to incorporate much more advanced ranking methods in which skills, attributes and qualifications, along with experience and location are conveyed as interchangeable values to provide sufficient flexibility for purpose, i.e. to abbreviate the selection cycle and meet pressing position appointment needs. Idealistic profiling of the imagined candidate(s) will thereby be subject to compromise. The healthcare demand intelligence system may require augmentation through additional class expressions and instance populations.

References

Chen, Y., Argentinis, J.D.E., Weber, G.: IBM watson: how cognitive computing can be applied to big data challenges in life sciences research. Clin. Ther. **38**(4), 688–701 (2016)

Forbes, D.E.: A Framework for Assistive Communications Technology in Cross-Cultural Healthcare. Curtin University (2013)

Freitas, A., Panisson, A.R., Hilgert, L., Meneguzzi, F., Vieira, R., Bordini, R.H.: Integrating ontologies with multi-agent systems through CArtAgO artifacts. In: 2015 IEEE/WIC/ACM International Conference on Web Intelligence and Intelligent Agent Technology (WI-IAT), Singapore: IEEE (2015)

Garanina, N.O., Sidorova, E., Bodin, E.V.: A multi-agent approach to unstructured data analysis based on domain-specific ontology. In: 22nd International Workshop on Concurrency, Specification and Programming, Warsaw, Poland: Citeseer (2013)

Gwynne, K., Lincoln, M.: Developing the rural health workforce to improve Australian Aboriginal and Torres Strait Islander health outcomes: a systematic review. Australian Health Review. http://www.publish.csiro.au/ah/AH15241 (2016)

Infections Persist, Pandemics Rule. The Spectator Australia. 22 Apr 2017. Available at https://spectator.com.au/2017/04/infections-persist-pandemics-rule/ (2017). Accessed 5 May 2017

Li, S., Mackaness, W.A.: A multi-agent-based, semantic-driven system for decision support in epidemic management. Health Inf. J. **21**(3), 195–208 (2015)

Li, L., Wu, B., Yang, Y.: Agent-based ontology integration for ontology-based applications. In: Proceedings of the 2005 Australasian Ontology Workshop. Sydney, Australia, Aust. Comput. Soc. Inc **58**, 53–59 (2005)

Monte-Alto, H., Biasão, A., Teixeira, L., Huzita, E.: Multi-agent applications in a context-aware global software development environment distributed computing and artificial intelligence. 265–272. Springer Berlin / Heidelberg (2012)

Oriche, A., Chekry, A., Khaldi, M.: Intelligent agents for the semantic annotation of educational resources. Int. J. Soft Comput. Eng. (IJSCE) **3**(5), 2231–2307 (2013)

Rosendal, M., Hartman, T.C.O., Aamland, A., van der Horst, H., Lucassen, P., Budtz-Lilly, A., Burton, C.: 'Medically unexplained' symptoms and symptom disorders in primary care: prognosis-based recognition and classification. BMC Fam. Pract. **18**(1), 18 (2017)

Simpkin, A.L., Schwartzstein, R.M.: Tolerating uncertainty—the next medical revolution? N. Engl. J. Med. **375**(18), 1713–1715 (2016)

Smalberger, C.: An employer demand intelligence framework. http://espace.library.curtin.edu.au/R?func=dbin-jump-full&local_base=gen01-era02&object_id=199399 (2013)

Teixeira, L.O., Huzita, E.: DiSEN-AlocaHR: A multi-agent mechanism for human resources allocation in a distributed software development environment. In: 11th International Conference in Distributed Computing and Artificial Intelligence. 227–234. Cham: Springer International Publishing (2014)

Thompson, S.: "Cultural competence in healthcare" email exchange with author Forbes 6 April (2017)

Trudgen, R.: Why warriors lie down and die: Towards an Understanding of Why the Aboriginal people of Arnhem Land Face the Greatest Crisis in health and education since European contact. Aboriginal Resource and Development Services, Darwin (2000)

Wang, M., Lee, C., Hsieh, K., Hsu, C., Acampora, G., Chang, C.: Ontology-based multi-agents for intelligent healthcare applications. J. Ambient Intell. Humanized Comput. **1**(2), 111–131 (2010)

Yang, K., Lo, A., Steele, R.: An Ontology-based Multi-Agent System for the Accommodation Industry. In: 13th Australasian World Wide Web Conference, AusWeb07, New South Wales, Australia, 30 Jun–4 Jul 2007. 193–205 (2007)

Ying, W., Ray, P., Lewis, L.: A methodology for creating ontology-based multi-agent systems with an experiment in financial application development. In: 46th Hawaii International Conference on, Wailea, Maui, Hawaii, USA, Sys. Sci. (HICSS), 7–10 Jan 2013. 3397–3406. IEEE (2013)

Chapter 9
Open Issue and Concluding Remarks

9.1 Introduction

Any serious research scientist will admit that we never know what there is to know in totality about a given problem and in consequence the 'best' route for finding a solution. Medical researchers and healthcare practitioners are to a great extent captive to convention for several good and yet not so good, reasons. All cultures to some extent contain flawed philosophies and practices in the context of providing societal value. In this book, we discuss western medical culture power-distance and unsatisfactory healthcare worker communications, notably placing patients at a disadvantage as a consequence of a lack of cultural competence. This communications deficit is not exclusive to the PPIE environment; it can be found as a pervasive influence in the broader philosophical beliefs and practices among professional healthcare groups and among patients. Among the apparently intractable areas of problem identification and solutions pathways, we find distinct division, with strong polarised views, in the epidemiological setting. Accompanying conflicts of opinion one harmful consequence is an increasingly hostile communications process predicament leading to stigmatization of the patient and patient communities within a specific but mysterious diagnosis and treatment research debate.

9.2 Employment and Service Communications

There are groups of patients suffering from what became known as a 'Lyme-like disease' (Collignon et al. 2016) referring to a tick/vector borne infection and resultant multiple debilitating co-conditions. This emotionally contentious divisive and somewhat confused topic is well-published throughout the world. It is not our purpose to explore it here as we shortly move on to the encompassing scope of

© Springer International Publishing AG 2018   99
D.E. Forbes et al., *Ontology Engineering Applications in Healthcare and Workforce Management Systems*, Studies in Systems, Decision and Control 123, DOI 10.1007/978-3-319-65012-8_9

Medically Unexplained Symptoms (MUS) in the overall context of inadequacies in communication for knowledge sharing.

We first point to our lack of shared knowledge, weaknesses in human level accord, i.e. agreement on principles of reasoning; and our inability to know everything we need to know, in significant quantitative and qualitative terms. To overcome encumbrances in our ability to contextually comprehend detailed domain concept relationships, to be able to comprehensively collate and analytically reason the data, and to arrive at and communicate higher quality decisions; will require intensive research, modelling and validation for ontology based multi-agent systems development to resolve.

The foregoing acts as segue to the deep and demanding philosophical argument about MUS. We are effectively addressing what has become known as 'Blame Game' communications as illuminated by Stone (2014). The article is a comprehensive attempt to reconcile divided patient—doctor perspectives, and to arrive at an equitable shared approach to solving a mystery which by default is caught up in medical convention. Stone (2014) concluded that it is challenging for patients with medically unexplained symptoms to cope. Without a diagnosis, they are struggling to be accepted as real patients with real illnesses and being blamed for their own distress. Deep feelings of worthlessness and shame can be experienced by all which can lead to defensive behaviour in medical consultations. It then can trigger anxious or even hostile feelings in their doctors. GPs can also feel a sense of hopelessness and frustration.

The article prompts us to pose the question "Is the prevalent MUS healthcare service impasse experienced by many professionals an illustration of the limitations of human mental capacity in collating and analysing relevant medical data?" Further, "Are we seeing a strong case for ICT intervention interpretation and decision support?"

For consideration of the views of authors who come from the psychiatric and psychology disciplines or from medical circles subscribing to the original philosophical ontology understanding of the human MUS condition as being 'all in the mind', we have reviewed the following papers, which we recommend as sources deserving of respect and a contributory value when developing or expanding machine ontology domain properties, relationships and contextual communications data:

- Explaining the unexplained? Overcoming the distortions of a dualist understanding of medically unexplained illness (Deary 2005)
- At the borders of medical reasoning: aetiological and ontological challenges of medically unexplained symptoms (Eriksen et al. 2013)
- Medically unexplained symptoms and the disease label (Jutel 2010).

Jutel (2010) explored the discursive construction of such symptoms in the medical literature and stated MUS are recast as a discrete category. This implies the infallibility of the physician and the relevance of the medical model in all circumstances. It transfers responsibility for the disorder to the patient in a way that may hinder resolution, and it ignores socio-historical practices that influence when and why patients consult a physician. In a further exposition of the 'infallibility' posture (Jutel 2010) reported a post mortem study which had revealed discrepancies in major diagnosis of 39% and of minor diagnosis in 50% of cases respectively. Jutel (2010) also referred to Lyme disease by stating that before its designation as a specific diagnosable condition, it was commonly labelled as atypical rheumatoid arthritis.

As a signpost to the Australian pathway for justifying a much more sophisticated, analytical, machine support system for responding to the healthcare service needs, from health professional recruitment cultural competence qualifications to cross cultural communications, we have identified the exceptional population engagement factors which strongly emphasize the importance of building greater patient centred equity and versatility in the PPIE environment.

The Multicultural Mental Health Australia (MHiMA) project funded by the Australian Government, Department of Health, provides a national focus for advice and support to providers and governments on mental health and suicide prevention for people from CALD backgrounds (The Multicultural Mental Health Australia (MHiMA) n.d.). In a solicited submission to the MHiMA Project consultation, in February 2016 a Joint submission was emailed from the Federation of Ethnic Communities' Councils of Australia (FECCA) and the National Ethnic Disability Alliance (NEDA) (2016).

With credible supporting data source references, the submission presented in two aspects i.e. cultural and linguistic diversity in Australia and humanitarian entrants as follows:

- Cultural and Linguistic Diversity in Australia: the Australian Bureau of Statistics reports that at 30 June 2014, 28.1% of Australia's estimated resident population was born overseas, that is, 6.6 million people. Over 4 million of these were born in non-English speaking countries.
- Humanitarian Entrants: a total of 199,765 humanitarian entrants have arrived in Australia between 2000 and 2014.3 Australia's current humanitarian intake constitutes 13,750 places and is set to increase to 16,250 places in 2017–2018 and 18,750 places in 2018–2019 financial year. In addition, Australia is in the process of resettling 12,000 Syrian and Iraqi refugees.

9.3 Concluding Commentary

Key points from Kelly (2015) reinforce our conclusion that we remain on a perpetual, intellectually demanding, journey of research into development of integrated systems employing cognitive computing, bringing together ontology work, merging and matching data systems, and intelligent agents to elevate human intelligence capabilities and benefits. In particular, we must endure to shape the effect of cognitive computing on work and employment. Like all technology, cognitive computing will change the nature of work done by people. It will assist us to perform tasks faster and more accurately. It will make many processes inexpensive and efficient. It will also do some things better than humans, which has been the case since the dawn of civilization. Given the exponential growth in knowledge, discovery and opportunity opened up by a Cognitive Era; there is every reason to believe that the human work will become ever more interesting, challenging and valuable. Societal controls and safeguards are equally important and needed, though such concerns are not unique to intelligent systems. Security questions for both individuals and institutions are assigned to every transformational technology, from automobiles to pharmaceuticals to mobile phones. These issues are vital and will remain so as cognitive technologies develop. They are fuelled especially by today's radical democratization of technology driven by the rapid spread of networks and the Cloud; and the accompanying desire for efficient cost reduction. The answer lies not in attempting to limit that democratization, but rather in embracing it while designing cognitive systems with privacy, security and human control integrated within it.

Reviewing the above excerpted key points from Kelly (2015) allows us to further conclude and draw from the work we have undertaken here, with three cogent statements:

- The EDI and CCHC domains are construed and as such are in combination examples from the latent pool of infinite permutations of societal pursuits in artificial intelligence or cognitive computing technology.
- Task based equitable cognitive competence in communications, regardless of the ethnic or work culture of human participants, represents a major goal as we face the multi-faceted challenges which place employment demands and healthcare service delivery at the forefront of public and private investment.
- Steady but disparate and segregated progress in domain specific ontologies exists; but more sophisticated large scale and greatly enriched contextually intelligent matched and merged systems are a priority for development; leading to far-reaching implementation of new working models—in our case in support of EDI and CCHC.

References

Collignon, P.J., Lum, G.D., Robson, J.M.B.: Does lyme disease exist in Australia? Med. J. Aust. **205**, 413–417 (2016). doi:10.5694/mja16.00824

Deary, V.: Explaining the unexplained? Overcoming the distortions of a dualist understanding of medically unexplained illness. J. Mental Health **14**, 213–221 (2005)

Eriksen, T.E., Kerry, R., Mumford, S., Lie, S.A.N., Anjum, R.L.: At the borders of medical reasoning: aetiological and ontological challenges of medically unexplained symptoms. Philos Ethics Humanit. Med. **8**, 11 (2013). doi:10.1186/1747-5341-8-11

Joint Submission from the Federation of Ethnic Communities' Councils of Australia (FECCA) and the National Ethnic Disability Alliance (NEDA) to MHiMA Project Consultation. Available at http://Fecca.org.au/Wp-Content/Uploads/2016/02/MHiMA-Project-Submission-to-MHA.pdf (2016). Accessed 4 Jun 2016

Jutel, A.: Medically unexplained symptoms and the disease label. Soc. Theory Health **8**, 229–245 (2010). doi:10.1057/sth.2009.21

Kelly, J.E., III.: Computing, cognition and the future of knowing—How humans and machines are forging a new age of understanding. IBM White Paper (2015)

Stone, L.: Blame, shame and hopelessness: medically unexplained symptoms and the 'heartsink' experience. Aust. Fam. Phys. **43**, 191–195 (2014)

The Multicultural Mental Health Australia (MHiMA) Available at http://www.mhima.org.au/. n.d. Accessed 12 Dec 2017

Printed in the United States
By Bookmasters